TennCare and Disproportionate Share Hospitals

Chinyere Ogbonna

University Press of America,® Inc.
Lanham · Boulder · New York · Toronto · Plymouth, UK

Copyright © 2007 by
University Press of America,® Inc.
4501 Forbes Boulevard
Suite 200
Lanham, Maryland 20706
UPA Acquisitions Department (301) 459-3366

Estover Road
Plymouth PL6 7PY
United Kingdom

Library of Congress Control Number: 2006934334
ISBN-13: 978-0-7618-3646-9 (paperback : alk. paper)
ISBN-10: 0-7618-3646-2 (paperback : alk. paper)

⊖™ The paper used in this publication meets the minimum
requirements of American National Standard for Information
Sciences—Permanence of Paper for Printed Library Materials,
ANSI Z39.48—1984

Dedication

This book is dedicated to my mom, Mabel Ogbonna, and my children, Nwachi, Chima and Chike McGruder.

Contents

Figures

Tables

Foreword

TennCare was developed as a bold strategy to simultaneously contain rapidly rising Medicaid costs and expand health insurance for a large uninsured population using a Medicaid Section 1115 Waiver. At the stroke of midnight on January 1, 1994, all of Tennessee's Medicaid population was moved into fully-capitated managed care plans. The initial savings from reduced inpatient hospital spending were sufficient to allow TennCare's rolls to expand by 50 percent immediately and the projected savings offered the possibility of near-universal coverage in the state. By the end of January, 1994 1.2 million TennCare beneficiaries were enrolled in one of 12 participating managed care plans (6 Health Maintenance Organizations and 6 Preferred provider Organizations). This was a remarkable achievement in a state that the year before had only eleven small HMOs enrolling a total of 216,000 Tennessee residents. By design, TennCare was used as an instrument to greatly accelerate managed care development in Tennessee.

The original waiver allowed the state to expand subsidized coverage to families with incomes to 400 percent of the Federal Poverty Line and unsubsidized coverage to individuals of any income. Federal funding supported these expansions in an era when many states were exploring health care reform and the Clinton Administration was supporting a sweeping overhaul of the nation's health care system based on competing managed care plans. The state financed its share of TennCare costs by, among other things, redirecting Disproportionate Share (DSH) Medicaid Payments from hospitals to the insurance program. Blue-Cross/ Blue-Shield, the state's dominant insurer was a critical anchor for the new program and it established an adequate physician network for its TennCare plan by requiring its contracted physicians to participate in TennCare in order to be eligible to participate in the state employee network. This requirement came to be known as the "cram-down" provision and was resented by many physicians.

From the start, the program was controversial. Concerns were raised about the program's costs, as well as poor risk and enrollment management. Provider opposition was intense as the program imposed managed care cost controls in a state that had previously experienced little managed care penetration. Some of the new health plans were provider-sponsored and most of these experienced significant learning-curve problems. In addition, the usual health policy schisms emerged. Liberals fought to protect and expand eligibility and benefits, and advocacy groups filed lawsuits to block cuts aimed at controlling costs. Conservatives considered the program too generous and opposed the subsidies and income transfers it entailed.

In 2000, the program began to unravel. Blue Cross blamed TennCare for loses and demanded that the state take back financial risk for the program. In 2002, the federal government refused to continue contributing to the cost of coverage expansions when the Section 1115 Waiver was renewed. During this same time period, managed care was losing control of health care costs nationwide as it evolved away from restricted networks, deep provider discounts and strict utilization controls, and several states that had implemented ambitious health care reforms were curtailing these programs in the face of relentless cost increases. Political support for TennCare was further eroded when Governor Dan Sundquist linked financing the program to an unpopular proposal to implement a state income tax. As Tennessee, along with the nation, slid into recession in 2001, TennCare was consuming 26 percent of the state's budget and there was a growing consensus for scaling-back the program. This was done by Governor Phil Bredesen and for all intents and purposes, the TennCare experiment in over. Despite its shortcomings, TennCare succeeded in significantly reducing Tennessee's uninsured population. By 1999, the program insured more than half-a-million individuals who did not qualify for Medicaid. In the early years, it also did a reasonable job of controlling cost increases. As a group, participating health plans were profitable until 1997.

The debate over the lessons of TennCare and the causes of its demise has been joined and is highly relevant for policy-makers today. In many respects, TennCare demonstrated both the potential and the limitations of state-level health care reform. Its implementation in a medium-sized state without an income tax was a remarkable achievement and demonstrates the potential for progressive policy-makers to take bold steps given favorable circumstances. However, as in many other states, large coverage expansions could not be sustained in Tennessee, suggesting the need for a strong federal role in future reforms.

Dr. Ogbonna has studied the TennCare program for many years and offers valuable insights concerning a key aspect of the program's financing, the diversion of DSH payments from hospitals to the insurance program. In this work, she explores the impact of this decision on Tennessee hospitals. As DSH payments offer a significant potential source of funds for future health care reforms aimed at expanding insurance coverage, her work should be of interest to policy-makers and health service managers alike.

Wayne Higgins, Ph.D.
Professor of Health Service Administration
Western Kentucky University

Preface

The recession and rising health care costs experienced by many states in United States have led to the enactment or a move towards the enactment of legislation that would reform the way that health care is provided for and paid for within their states. The health care system reform plan implemented in the state of Tennessee on Jan 1, 1994 is known as TennCare. The main objectives of the reform plan were to control the rapidly rising costs of the state's Medicaid program and extend health insurance coverage to most Tennesseans that did not have access to employer sponsored or other government sponsored health insurance. Beneficiaries enrolled in competing, state chartered managed care organizations that are responsible for providing a broad range of inpatient, outpatient, and preventive services, for which they are reimbursed on a capitation basis by the state at a rate based on a statewide global budget for health care. This book describes the design, rationale, benefits and problems of TennCare as well as interest groups reaction and the policy actors involved in implementation of the state reform. The analytic focus of the book is on the effects of TennCare reimbursement on disproportionate share hospitals in Tennessee. All the hospitals within the state of Tennessee were included in the study for this book. The non-disproportionate share hospitals served as controls for the study. Data spanning a ten year period were obtained from these hospitals. The data pertained to admissions/discharges, average median daily census and profit. Statistical analyses were performed on the data for the disproportionate and non-disproportionate share hospitals.

Results of the study indicate that TennCare implementation did not have adverse effects on average median daily census and admissions/discharges of disproportionate share hospitals. But TennCare implementation appeared to have an adverse impact on profit, of these hospitals.

The book is targeted towards Political science and Health care management/policy professionals and students, as well as individuals who are interested in learning more about the innovative TennCare program instituted by the State of Tennessee. Hopefully the book will generate interest in exploring different strategies for managing the costs of health care (at both State and Federal level), while ensuring coverage for the majority of the population.

Organization of the Book

The first chapter of the book focuses on introducing the subject matter and on the significance of the TennCare study on public policy making with regards to health care issues. Chapter 2 expands on the TennCare reform issue and also includes more review of literature pertaining to health care and policy issues.

Chapter 3 depicts the methodology utilized in this study. This chapter describes the research design and limitations of the research design. The chapter also focuses on the definition of the population under study, as well as on survey and data collection protocol.

Chapter 4 comprises of data analysis and also includes statistical analysis and brief discussion of the results. The basis for accepting or rejecting the null hypotheses is included too. Chapter 5 interprets and summarizes results of the study, while discussing implications for further research and future public policy.

Acknowledgments

I would like to acknowledge the support and guidance provided throughout this process by Dr Wayne Higgins. I am profoundly grateful for the encouragement and assistance provided by Mr. Ross Nordin who was invaluable in helping make this book a reality. Mr. Lonnell Matthews of the Tennessee Department of Health was instrumental in providing the hospital statistics data. I am very grateful for the unconditional love of my children and finally I would like to thank my parents and especially my mom, Mabel Ogbonna for her indefatigable encouragement and love.

Chapter 1
Introduction

The health care system in United States is uniquely different from that of other nations, in that it is substantially more costly than any foreign system. A 1998 OECD[1] health data report indicates that the health care system in United States is the most expensive, outstripping by far the health care expenditures of any other country.[2] Studies also indicate that a large percentage of the United States population is uninsured, more than any other industrialized nation.[3] The problem of increasing health care costs have led to different strategies, (both at the federal and different state levels) aimed at controlling the growth of these health care costs. The wide spread adoption of managed care with its austere and strict reimbursement rates and low national inflation rate, have considerably slowed the rate of growth of medical spending. Despite this, a new government study indicates that health care expenditures would soon begin to increase and there is the real possibility that it would double within the next decade.[4] Therefore it is obvious that tangible ways of keeping health care costs down are necessary so as to avoid the possibility of overwhelming the economy of the nation.

Different states have enacted or are making moves towards the enactment of legislation that would reform the way that health care is provided and paid for within their Medicaid programs. The health care system reform plan implemented by the state of Tennessee on 1st January 1994, is known as TennCare. TennCare was implemented by the state of Tennessee in an effort to curb rapidly rising Medicaid health care costs while simultaneously providing greater coverage for previously uninsured patients.

This book is structured towards examining the effects of TennCare reimbursement on Tennessee hospitals that serve a disproportionate share of low income individuals. The study utilized for the purpose of this book, will focus on the effects of TennCare implementation on patient daily census, admissions/discharges, and financial performance or profit of these hospitals.

It is necessary to briefly trace the origin and historical development of health services in United States. This will provide some sort of background on the issue of increasing health care costs both at the federal and state levels.

A Brief History of the Financing, Costing and Economics of Health Care in the United States

In the United States, prior to the turn of the 20th century, individuals were expected to pay for the costs of their medical services. These services were usually provided by both physicians and nurses. Those that could not afford to pay for private physicians and medications had to utilize charitable institutions. These institutions were established as voluntary, nonprofit corporations that provided charity health care for indigent patients.

The beginning of the 20th century saw the development of city/county hospitals, which were established by local governments to provide care for indigent patients in their areas or locales. These indigent patients could not pay for their own care nor obtain the services of the charity hospitals.[5] These hospitals were usually large acute care facilities with busy clinics and emergency rooms with close connections to local government ambulance services, police department and other community services. During the same period, state governments also began to assume responsibility for the care of the insane.[6]

After World War II there was a surge in health care costs, with resultant increase in development and the variety of health insurance plans. The post-war period saw the development of community based non-profit Blue Cross/Blue Shield plans,[7] and labor union health and welfare trust funds. These funds were established as a result of benefit negotiations for union members. During this period, private for profit commercial insurance companies increased their scope of efforts for the benefit of their beneficiaries. Their beneficiaries included both individuals and large groups of employees. It was within this period that different and large government sponsored and publicly managed insurance health care plans evolved, such as Medicare and Medicaid.[8]

The growth or increase in these health insurance plans seemed to occur in tandem with development of private medical practitioners, city and state government hospitals, voluntary nonprofit hospitals as well as military and veteran hospitals. This variety in the provision of health care seemed suited for United states with its wide diversity of people and situations.[9]

The period encompassing 1945 through 1970 was rife with developments in United States health care.[10] These developments were governed by mutual interests between insurers and providers who formed a sort of coalition that allowed for flow of funds from payers of care to insurers, providers and suppliers of health care.[11] These funds helped promote scientific progress in the field of medicine.[12] After 1970 there were obvious signs of deteriorating United States economy, while simultaneously health care costs were rapidly increasing. The increasing health care costs were spurred by great strides in intricate andcostly biotechnological development and the public's desire to utilize expensive most advanced treatment and diagnostic techniques. Thus deterioration of United States economy and rapid increase in health care expenditures clashed with the need for biotechnological development and the public's desire for advanced diagnostic techniques and treatment. This was a major factor in spiraling health care costs. The major payers i.e. government and business, tried to stem the growth of health care funding. This led to an uneasy relationship between insurers and providers of care thus straining their alliance, while opening the health care sector to immense political and economic change.[13] Bodenheimer and Grumbach indicated that:

> As the payers limited which insurers and providers would receive payments, competition intensified within the health care industry with the big-large insurers. large hospitals, and large physician groups gaining ascendancy over the small. Selective contracting gives payers a great deal of power because they can deny contracts with insurers and providers who fail to keep costs down. The heightened power of the payers has led to a new relationship between insurers and providers. First, HMOs merge insurers and providers into one organization; thus, insurers owning HMOs also function as providers of care. Second, within insurer-controlled HMOs, the insurers play the role of managers while the true providers-hospitals and physicians -are the direct producers of medical services. In some cases, HMOs own hospitals and employ physicians. In other cases, HMOS determine which hospitals and physicians will receive their patients and how much those providers will be paid.[14]

Therefore providers no longer have full autonomy in determining their fees. This lack of full autonomy has spawned a system where insurers now virtually call the shots in determining how much providers can be paid for their services.

There are different participants, in the trillion-dollar health care industry, but Thomas Bodenhimer and Kevin Grumbach emphasize that modern day health care stage is comprised of four major actors. These actors are: 1) The payers who supply the money to pay for utilized health care. The payers would include individuals[15] that utilize health care services, businesses that pay for their employees' health insurance and government since it provides payment for care through public programs such as Medicare and Medicaid; 2) The insurers who take money from payers, assume risk and then pay providers when policy holders need medical care. So insurers basically receive money from payers and utilize some of the money to reimburse providers;[16] 3) Providers who are the individuals or organizations that actually provide the health care; 4) Suppliers would refer to the pharmaceutical and medical supply industries that provide health care equipments, supplies and medications utilized by providers in treating patients.[17] These different participants are interconnected in the insurance, management and provision of health services. It is necessary to understand the interrelationship between these participants so as to have a basic comprehension of the health care process within United States.

There is an underlying tension between payers/insurers of health care and members of the health care industry i.e. providers and suppliers of health care.

Whenever the payer or insurer spends money for health care it represents income to the health care industry. Payers wish to contain their costs, while providers and suppliers of health care wish to see an increase in the amount of money spent on health care.

It is difficult to specify with any degree of certainty a particular proven or consistent modus operandi of health care in United States. It would seem that new and different ideas predominate for a while within the health care field but with passage of time, these ideas appear not to work nor produce any sort of solution to the problem of providing quality and cost efficient health care. Hence the general perspective is that the health care field goes through periods of evolution in the process of trying to attain an optimum goal, whereby every citizen would have quality health coverage at a reasonable cost. The changes undergone by the health care field in United States would include shifting from payment of services rendered to buying into indemnity type insurance plans (which pay providers on a fee for service basis), to federal government involvement in paying for health insurance plans. Currently there is an emphasis on Managed Care plans that advocate some sort of implicit rationing of health care in the pursuit of reduced health care costs. All these changes came about when it seemed that the former way of payment and provision of services did not appear to provide adequate health coverage at a reasonable price.

These changes or revolutions could be likened to Thomas Kuhn's assertions about scientific revolutions.[18] The author's assertions imply that if a paradigm can no longer solve "problems," then there is the tendency for the paradigm to be replaced with another. In other words the old paradigm is seen as being "insufficient" and this consequently leads to "scientific revolutions." These revolutions are considered the result of a "crisis."
According to the author:

> The transition from a paradigm in crisis to a new one from which a new tradition of normal science can emerge is far from a cumulative process, one achieved by an articulation or extension of the old paradigm. Rather it is a reconstruction of the field from new fundamentals, a reconstruction that changes some of the field's most elementary theoretical generalizations as well as many of its paradigm methods and applications. During the transition period there will be a large but never complete overlap between the problems that can be solved by the old and by the new paradigm. But there will also be a decisive difference in the modes of solution. When the transition is complete, the profession will have changed its view of the field, its methods, and its goals.[19]

The above process could be visualized within context of the health care industry, whereby the industry appears to have gone through so many transitions in trying to find a cost effective means of providing health care. These transitions would include as mentioned before, focusing on indemnity type plans and then shifting focus from such plans to managed care plans. The transitions and changes could also be perceived in terms of reimbursement, which has run the gamut from reimbursement based on charges, to reimbursement based on hospital costs, to Diagnosis Related Group (DRG) reimbursement[20] methods and to what is currently most common--reimbursement based on predetermined rates by managed care organizations.

There is no single or easily described American system of health care, instead there are four models or subsystems of health care in America, each of which serve a different group of individuals. Accordingly these systems serve the following different groups:

(1) Regularly employed, middle-income families with continuous programs of health insurance coverage; (2) poor, unemployed (or underemployed) families without continuous health insurance coverage; (3) active-duty military personnel and their dependents; and (4) veterans of United States military service.[21]

A similar view of the United States frame work for health insurance can be broken down into three categories which reflect to some extent the employment status of individuals in the insurance program. These categories would include: Voluntary Health Insurance (VHI), which is usually private insurance that covers current industrial employees; Social Health Insurance (SHI), which indicates participation in a government entitlement program that is linked to prior employment and finally; Public Welfare programs which are for individuals that do not have employment, have low income employment or are unable to gain employment due to disability.[22]

These above two schema for classifying the United States health system recognize the significance of no insurance for the unemployed or underemployed. For purposes of this book much emphasis would be placed on the poor, employed/underemployed or unemployed families without continuous health insurance coverage. This is because Medicaid is a government sponsored insurance program for indigent individuals and TennCare was implemented to address the failings of Medicaid in providing widespread insurance coverage for its indigent population without crippling the economy of the state of Tennessee.

Background on Medicare and Medicaid

Medicare was instituted as part of Social Security Amendments of 1965, which established two separate but coordinated health insurance plans for persons aged 65 or older. The first part is know as part A of Medicare and it is the compulsory program of hospital insurance (HI), which provides hospital insurance for qualified individuals. The second part is B, and it is a voluntary program of Supplementary Medical Insurance (SMI). The SMI was intended to complement the HI program. As such it provides payment for physician's services, outpatient services as well as rural and home health visits for individuals without Part A. Medicare was amended in 1972 to provide coverage for certain severely disabled persons under the age of 65 and to individuals suffering from end stage renal disease. This was in addition to providing general coverage for individuals over the age of 60.[23]

Medicare was operated initially as a fee for service plan for physicians and related services. Hospital reimbursement at the same time was based on any reasonable costs incurred in provision of covered care to Medicare patients. But with increasing costs, reimbursement format was changed in 1983, to prospective payment system, where rates were determined on a case basis, using diagnosis-related groups (DRGs) to classify cases for reimbursement.[24] The DRG is a Yale University-derived system of classification for 383 inpatient hospital services that are based on principal diagnosis, secondary diagnosis, surgical procedures, sex, age and the presence of complications. This DRG classification is therefore utilized as a basis for compensating hospitals and other providers.[25] The cost of Medicare had been increasing, so the Tax Equity and Fiscal Responsibility Act of 1982 (TEFRA) was implemented. This law set limits on hospital costs reimbursements at the per case level and also limited the annual rate of increase for Medicare's reasonable costs per discharge.[26] Major components of the law, included revisions to the Medicare law to encourage growth in number of Health Maintenance Organizations (HMO) and other comprehensive medical plans that enroll Medicare beneficiaries.[27]

Medicaid was instituted into law as a Title XIX program of the Social Security Act on July 30, 1965.[28] Prior to enactment of Medicaid, states and local governments took care of the poor in their respective locales. In some instances doctors donated their services or assessed indigent patients charges for services on a sliding scale. But with enactment of Medicaid, the program became part of existing federal-state welfare structure.[29] Thus Medicaid was initially planned as a medical care extension of federally funded income maintenance programs for the poor with a focus on provision of care for dependent children and their mothers.[30] Since Medicaid is welfare medicine, it has no entitlement features, so recipients must prove their eligibility according to their income. Medicaid eligibility criteria and services provided are complex and vary considerably among states. Services can change within a state during the year and also one [31]can be eligible for certain services in one state but would not be eligible in another state. This is because the states have the option of choosing their criteria for eligibility. There is a great deal of variability within state standards for income and asset levels for cash assistance and medical eligibility. It is also within authority of states to determine scope of services provided.[32]

Since its inception the Medicaid program has been operated as a vendor payment system, which was designed to provide more effective medical care for individuals that needed it. This was to be achieved through improved standards of care, liberal eligibility rules and increased federal matching under a formula with no limit.[33]

Medicaid is welfare medicine whereas Medicare is a form of social health insurance (SHI). Within that context Medicaid is a transfer payment 'in kind" which implies that medical services are provided as a welfare benefit instead of cash. Cash subsides are also provided for welfare recipients to pay for their living expenses, although their medical benefits are paid directly to the providers so as to make it impossible for recipients to spend the money on expense items other than health care.[34]

Social health insurance (SHI) on the other hand, is not charity but entitlement program. In that regards it is a right earned by individuals in the course of their employment. Payroll tax is utilized in funding SHI programs, for example social security is funded by payroll tax which is divided between the worker and employer. Social health insurance programs are supposed to provide members of society with protection against hazards that are so widespread as to be considered risks that individuals cannot afford to deal with on their own. Therefore eligibility in SHI is derived from contributions that have been made to the program and benefits are statutory rights not based on need, so recipients are entitled to benefits of SHI.[35]

Medicaid spending is one of the fastest growing areas of state spending. In order to try and control costs, different strategies were utilized by different state governments. Such strategies included prepaid managed health care, utilization review, case management, reimbursement via diagnosis related group (DRG) and new services for elderly, disabled and AIDS stricken individuals. Currently the focus is on shifting Medicaid funding from federal to state budgets while encouraging states to pattern their systems after Health Maintenance Organizations (HMOs).[36] TennCare was patterned after HMOs,[37] in that the plan is fundamentally Medicaid being operated as a managed care program.

There has been no particular study to date that has focused on effects of TennCare on disproportionate share hospitals. The crucial aspect of this book it its focus on the effects of TennCare implementation on patient average daily census, admissions/discharges and financial performance or profit of hospitals that serve a disproportionate share of low income individuals. These effects would be compared with patient average daily census, admissions/discharges and profit of non-disproportionate share hospitals in Tennessee.

TennCare is structured so that managed care companies take over management of former Medicaid patients that are now insured under the health reform system. With managed care companies enrolling Medicaid beneficiaries in the state, there is possibility of undermining the infrastructure that provided indigent care in the past especially since the reimbursement rates for TennCare patients are very low. This is because the hospitals that treat indigent patients require the Medicaid reimbursement to stay viable. But with enrollment of Medicaid patients in managed care programs and subsequent lower reimbursement rates of managed care the viability of these hospitals could be threatened. On the other hand, TennCare extended insurance coverage to many who were previously uninsured, presumably reducing indigent care burden on disproportionate share hospitals.[38] The managed care plans may also redirect patients among hospitals, since the enrolled have to choose hospitals that are part of the managed care plans. Thus, the overall impact of TennCare on disproportionate share hospitals need to be studied in determining future public policy issues relating to health care insurance.[39] It is also necessary to study the general effects of managed care

reform plans on disproportionate share hospitals and hospitals in general. This
study would thus shed some light on whether implementation of TennCare un-
dermines the financial infrastructure of hospitals that serve a disproportionate
amount of indigent patients. It would also determine if hospital utilization and
admissions/discharges are affected by TennCare implementation. The research
would be a mostly descriptive quantitative study that would determine how
TennCare implementation has affected the performance and utilization of these
hospitals.

Basis for TennCare Implementation

In the late 1980s and early 1990s, majority of the states in United States were in
the middle of a health care crisis exacerbated by recession and rising health care
costs. In the light of this situation many states implemented various health care
reforms. By mid 1990s, eight states had enacted laws that were geared toward
the goal of ensuring access to medical care for all of their citizens.[40] Except for
Hawaii, none of the states that have enacted universal coverage laws since 1993
have fully implemented them[41]. These states have not been able to do so because
of a federal law, namely the Employee Retirement Income Security act (ERISA)
of 1974, which bars states from requiring employers to offer health benefits. In
order that employers are required to provide health insurance coverage for their
employees, a state would have to win a congressional exemption from ERISA[42],
and only Hawaii was granted such an exemption because its Prepaid Health Care
Act was passed before ERISA became law. Apart from the obstacle posed by
ERISA, any attempt to achieve universal coverage and tighter cost control must
be coordinated with the Medicare program.

By early 1990s, the states were being encouraged to try new ways of financing and delivering health or medical care. This was shown by willingness of the
federal government to waive Medicaid requirements that prevented innovation
by states. Tennessee took advantage of this option.

Like most of the other states, Tennessee faced major health care system
problems. Medicaid spending and the number of enrollees in the state had grown
so rapidly in past years[43] that health costs for enrollees, were starting to threaten
financial stability of the state's treasury. At the beginning of 1993, several years
of burgeoning growth in Tennessee Medicaid expenditures had created a budget
crisis that affected the entire state government.[44] The increase in the number of
eligible Medicaid recipients as well as health care cost inflation had nearly tri-
pled health care expenditures in just five years. As in so many other states,
Medicaid was the second largest and fastest growing item in Tennessee's
budget.[45] In fact cost of the program had grown so steeply that it threatened the
viability of all other functions of Tennessee state government. Out of all the
states in the union, Tennessee was ranked 11th in terms of Medicaid enrollee
numbers and was 17th in total Medicaid expenditures.[46] This was despite the fact
that an estimated 470,000 Tennesseans were without health insurance. Medicaid

growth had exceeded the ability of the state to sustain through normal methods of state revenue generation.[47] The state could no longer afford the uncontrollable expansion in Medicaid program costs, so a better solution had to be found.

In Tennessee, as with other states in United States, the largest portion of health care expenditures goes to the hospitals. Total Medicaid costs in Tennessee grew from approximately $692 million in fiscal year (FY) 1988-1989 to almost $2.7 billion in FY 1993-1994, while number of recipients increased from 540,000 to almost 1 million. The compounded average annual growth in number of enrollees was 13.1%, and the average cost per enrollee increased at a rate of 7.4% per year.[48] Despite the fact that Tennessee had a high Medicaid eligibility standard,[49] as mentioned previously, it ranked 11th when compared with other states in terms of Medicaid enrollees and ranked 17th in total Medicaid expenditures.[50] Tennessee also ranked 44th nationally in per capita income, but relative amount of money spent on hospital care in Tennessee increased when measured as a percent of total state per capita income. In 1973, Tennessee was ranked 4th in United States, but by 1981, the state's rate of increase had risen to number 1 in the country.[51] The increasing health costs incurred by the state were not resulting in increased quality of care or adequate access to care.[52] In addition a lot of needy people such as the working poor and the uninsured were excluded totally from public health assistance under Medicaid with no other available health insurance option. Although about 70 % of the uninsured had jobs or were dependents of employed persons, medical benefits were usually not offered at their jobs, and their wages were generally too low to pay for high premiums usually charged insured people that were not part of a large employee group. Therefore it would seem more beneficial to these workers to lose their jobs so as to be qualified for Medicaid thus discouraging indigent individuals from taking employment due to fear of losing their Medicaid benefits.[53] The high cost of medical and preventive care, in most instances led to non-utilization of preventive care or early treatment of conditions, and this neglect sometimes resulted in delayed and more expensive treatment for non-insured patients.[54]

In view of the problems faced by Tennessee, the then Governor, Ned McWherter, upon assuming office had managed to keep costs down by utilizing "creative financing" techniques. These techniques included provider taxes repaid through Disproportionate-Share Hospital (DSH) payments and other enhanced provider payments. These tactics were used to induce hospitals and nursing homes to fund some of the state's share of Medicaid Costs. This practice was fundamental in bringing about an increase in federal medical assistance percentage from 67.6 to about 83.1 percent during initial years of McWherter's administration, while simultaneously keeping Tennessee's medical spending down. The state thus had managed to hold down increase in its general revenue fund appropriations for Medicaid to less than 25 percent, despite the fact that the program's budget increased threefold during this period.[55]

Under federal law, when determining payment rates for inpatient hospital care, state Medicaid programs are required to "take into account the situation of hospitals that serve a disproportionate number of low income patients with special needs." This requirement is known as the Medicaid disproportionate share hospital (DSH) payment adjustment.[56] The Boren Amendment as established in (OBRA) Omnibus Budget Reconciliation Acts of 1980 and 1981, was legislation that brought into place the DSH program. This piece of legislation tried to maintain access to health care by mandating that states should consider special payment needs for hospitals that serve a large portion of Medicaid and uninsured patients. The reason was that hospitals that render high volumes of care to low income individuals usually lose money due to low Medicaid reimbursement rates.[57] These hospitals were also losing money because they generally provided high volumes of care to indigent patients and therefore had high levels of uncompensated care. Usually such hospitals with large caseloads of low-income patients generally have low private caseloads, thus making it harder for the hospitals to shift cost of uncompensated care to privately insured patients.[58]

The DSH payment legislation was enacted in the early 1980s but the different states did not really pick up on benefits of utilizing it, till beginning of 1990s. The DSH expenditures soared in the 1990s and by 1996, they accounted for one out of every eleven dollars spent on Medicaid.[59]

By early 1993, new federal laws designed to curb utilization of "Creative financing" techniques were being implemented.

The most important of these laws is the 1991 federal law know as Medicaid Voluntary Contribution and Provider Specific Tax Amendments of 1991 (P.L. 101-234).[60] The body of this law has requirements that would virtually eliminate provider donations as well as restrict provider taxes. As such, the 1991 law contained several restrictions for money that would be eligible for federal matching funds, thus making provider donations technically impossible, while at the same time bringing about a restriction in provider taxes. The federal Medicaid requirements were also changed so as to eliminate federal match for voluntary provider donations. The law was directly related to flagrant abuse of DSH payments and as such it was intended to regulate the way that states generated funds that would be utilized for attracting matching federal Medicaid funding.[61]

Key provisions of the law included: 1) Banning provider donations; 2) limitation of provider taxes so that provider tax revenues could not exceed 25 percent of each individual state's share of Medicaid expenditures; 3) imposition of provider tax criteria so that taxes were "broad based" and providers were not "held harmless",[62] and 4) capping DSH payments at about 1992 levels.[63]

The restrictions brought about by enactment of the 1991 law may be summarized as follows: Health care-related taxes that are eligible for federal matching funds must be broad-based, imposed uniformly and include all members of a class, such as all inpatient hospitals, all physicians or all HMOs and prepaid entities; taxes cannot make up more than 25 percent of a state's share of Medicaid; and taxes cannot also contain a "hold harmless" provision, which guarantees that health care providers will have the tax that they paid returned to them.[64]

It was difficult for states to establish tax and donation programs that complied with the 1991 law. Thus this law subsequently curtailed DSH payment growth and forced many states to restructure DSH financing and look for other ways of keeping their medical budget in balance.[65]

Prior to enactment of the 1991 law, utilization of "Creative financing" techniques by different states was possible simply because in 1985, Health Care Financing Administration (HCFA), started allowing states to include voluntary provider donations in calculation of federal matching payments under Medicaid. This made it possible for any individual state to collect voluntary provider donations to fund its Medicaid program. In Tennessee, this donation would be matched by the federal government at slightly better than two to one. These tactics were utilized to induce hospitals and nursing homes to fund part of the state's share of Medicaid costs, since they would receive higher Medicaid reimbursements in return.[66] Around 1980s, some states began to adopt provider tax programs, which operated along the same lines as the voluntary provider donation programs. These programs were of great financial benefit for the states that utilized them.[67] Each dollar of revenue raised from either a tax or donation program, could bring in one to four federal financial participation (FFP) dollars depending on the state's federal matching rate.[68] The following is an example of how a Medicaid DSH program worked prior to the 1991 Law:

(1) The state receives $20 million from a provider, in donation or tax.

(2) Since DSH payments are match able Medicaid expenses, the federal government can reimburse the state anywhere from 50 to 80 percent of the DSH payment, depending on the state's federal matching rate. Assuming the rate for this state is 50 percent, the federal government would then reimburse the state half of the $20 million and that would be $10 million.

(3) The state then makes a DSH payment back to the provider as a lump sum payment or as an increase in Medicaid reimbursement rate. In this case the state makes a $22 million DSH payment to the same provider that made the donation of $20 million. Thus the provider has earned $2 million in DSH payments while the state is short $2 million of the matching federal fund.

(4) The deal is concluded with the provider receiving $2 million extra in DSH payments, while the state had received $8 million (i.e. $10 million minus $2 million, it had to pay for DSH), in federal money without having to spend any of its own funds. The federal government has thus paid $10 million in DSH payments, whereas only $2 million of it was paid to DSH provider, while the state kept the balance.[69]

Such tactics were responsible for overwhelming growth in Medicaid DSH payment/utilization, and subsequent percentage increase of federal medical assistance from 67.6% to about 83.1%. Therefore it was possible for different states to control individual increases in their respective general fund appropriations for Medicaid, despite almost a threefold increase in general Medicaid budget. The Medicaid DSH payments thus made it possible to spend tax and donation revenues, especially since DSH payments were not subjected to the

Medicare upper payment limit. So states could make practically unlimited DSH payments while earning FFP dollars in the process.[70]

Starting from Oct. 1, 1992, a state's disproportionate-share payment[71] could not exceed 12 percent of its total Medicaid budget, but states above that limit could continue at their current percentage, while states below that limit could not surpass 12 percent. Thus enactment of this law made it mandatory for more than 30 states that had engaged in this type of funding to change the way that their Medicaid programs were funded.[72] This law thus curbed as well as changed the way that states could generate funds to attract matching Medicaid federal dollars.

Due to restrictions of the 1991 law, states then turned to intergovernmental transfer[73] (IGT) programs as their primary revenue source for their DSH programs.[74] Under these programs states would transfer funds from public institutions such as state psychiatric facilities, university hospitals and county and metropolitan hospitals to state Medicaid agency. The state would then make DSH payment back to these facilities while collecting federal matching Medicaid dollars in the process.[75] Since the IGT mechanism was billed as DSH payments to public facilities, it had the added advantage (over provider tax and donation programs) of preserving federal dollars for local and state institutions.[76] But, depending on the specifics of a program, private hospitals could be completely excluded under an IGT-financed DSH program.[77]

Implementation of the 1991 law curtailed DSH spending growth, but emergence of these IGT programs were of concern to federal policy makers. Policy makers questioned the appropriateness of DSH payments in certain circumstances, and they were especially concerned that some states were making DSH payments to facilities that were not large Medicaid providers.[78] Policy makers were also concerned that some other states utilized DSH payments which over compensated providers for unreimbursed costs incurred in caring for Medicaid and indigent patients. Thus some providers were getting DSH payments that exceeded the revenue that they received for rendering care to Medicaid patients.[79] In a nutshell, federal policy makers did not believe that DSH payments were being utilized for the intended purpose of helping safety-net providers. Instead they believed that DSH payments were being used to help general state financing.

In fact a 1993 survey of 39 states utilizing DSH programs indicated that 33 percent of their DSH funds were retained by the states rather than being paid to disproportionate-share hospitals.[80]

To address these issues, Congress included the following provisions to OBRA in 1993:

1) In order for a hospital to receive DSH payments, it should have a Medicaid use rate of at least 1 percent: 2) A single hospital could not receive total DSH payments that exceeded the unreimbursed costs of providing inpatient care to Medicaid and uninsured (Charity care) patients. These limits were effective in 1994 for most public hospitals and in 1995 for private hospitals.[81]

The provisions contained in the 1991 and 1993 laws, were critical in spurring different states to explore different avenues of managing their Medicaid programs, since they could no longer depend on DSH payment windfall. Thus several of the states have enacted or are in the process of enacting reforms in the way that their Medicaid or public health care insurance programs are administered. As of January 1995, ten states had gotten waivers from Health Care Financing Administration (HCFA),82 to reform the[82] administration of their health care programs especially Medicaid. These states included Arizona, Florida, Hawaii, Kentucky, Ohio, Oregon, Rhode Island, South Carolina and Tennessee. Six other states also had waiver submissions with HCFA. These six states included Delaware, Illinois, Louisiana, Massachusetts, Missouri and New Hampshire. Ten other states were considering waiver submissions, and these states included California, Connecticut, Kansas, Maryland, Nevada, New Jersey, New York, Oklahoma, Texas and Washington.[83] These states hoped to achieve autonomy in the way that they managed their Medicaid programs. They were hoping that this autonomy would be utilized in developing cost-sharing provisions or cost reduction techniques, such as shifting of Medicaid enrollees from a fee for service system to that of a managed care system.[84] This shift would supposedly result in savings to states that choose to undertake this route. Therefore this shift had the most impact on states that have tried to reform their Medicaid programs.[85]

After implementation of the 1991 and 1993 laws, Tennessee was faced with the possibility of losing $494 million in federal matching funding. Governor McWherter had to act so as to circumvent the crisis that could result from loss of matching federal funding.[86] The state could not afford to wait for a national health system reform to address the financial and access problems posed by Medicaid.[87] It was then necessary to formulate a different policy that would take into account problems facing the state with regards to increasing Medicaid costs and uninsured population.

These specific problems faced by Tennessee in managing its health care had to be taken into account when structuring a reform program or plan. Drastic reductions in coverage did not seem like a feasible solution since a large number of Tennessee's indigent population were already not insured under Medicaid.[88] So it was necessary to consider fundamental reform of the Medicaid program.

According to McWherter (1993), the state of Tennessee considered three policy options and they were as follows:

1) Substantial annual tax increase: This was not a fiscally or politically tenable option as Tennessee had not been a very wealthy state. Moreover Tennessee's constitution prohibits a state income tax. The state had tried to raise health care funds by levying a 6.7% broad-based tax on hospitals and other professional services. But health care organizations vigorously opposed this idea and the federal government restricted this method for increasing federal contributions to state Medicaid programs. The resultant decrease in federal funds made the state's financial crisis worse.

2) Massive reduction in reimbursement rates and in provision of healthcare services: This would also be impractical as these reductions would not solve the ultimate problem of high health costs. It would instead encourage cost shifting to insured or private pay patients reduce access of Medicaid recipients to health care services and also shift the site of these services from preventive or ambulatory clinics to more expensive hospital outpatient departments or emergency departments.

3)Fundamental health care reform: This seemed to be Tennessee's only realistic option and this would include major reform of both health care delivery system and financing system.[89]

On April 8, 1993 the then democratic governor of Tennessee, Governor Ned McWherter announced the broad outline of TennCare program. The overall general goals of the program being the following: Global budgeting, Standard benefit package, Pooling of purchasing power, Managed care, Incentives for preventive care, Elimination of inappropriate welfare benefits, Cost sharing, Quality control, and the elimination of class distinctions.

TennCare would hopefully assure cost neutrality for the federal government and also reduce health care costs for all levels of government from what they would have been under the Medicaid system. Former Governor Ned McWherter believed that TennCare would expand coverage to virtually every uninsured person in the state without reduction of services or increase in taxes. Instead this goal would be achieved by utilizing proposed cost savings that would be gotten from managing Medicaid as a managed care program. Implementation of TennCare needed approval from Health Care Financing Administration (HCFA) and waiving of key regulations governing Medicaid programs. Governor Ned McWherter submitted TennCare proposal to HCFA as a section 1115 research and demonstration waiver request on June 16 1993.

On November 18, 1993 after protracted negotiations involving the White House and Department of Health and Human Services (DHHS), Clinton Administration granted Tennessee a waiver that would allow it to provide health insurance for 1.5 million poor and uninsured people. Under TennCare proposal the state will shift 1 million Medicaid recipients into private managed care plans that will compete for patients across 12 regions of the state.[90]

Description of the Study

The crucial aspect of this book is the study that attempts to measure or determine the effects of TennCare reimbursement on disproportionate share hospitals. It will thus focus on effects of TennCare's implementation on patient average daily census, admissions/discharges and on financial performance or profit of these hospitals. These effects would be compared with average daily census, admissions/discharges and profit for other hospitals in Tennessee.

TennCare is structured so that managed care companies now take over management of former Medicaid patients that are now insured under the reform system. With managed care companies enrolling Medicaid beneficiaries in the state, there is the possibility of undermining the infrastructure that provided indigent care in the past. On the other hand, TennCare extended insurance coverage to many who were previously uninsured, presumably reducing indigent care burden on disproportionate share hospitals. Managed care plans may also redirect patients among hospitals, thereby possibly redirecting patients away from DSH. Thus, the overall impact of TennCare on disproportionate share hospitals is an important public policy issue that needs to be studied. The study will thus address questions or issues pertaining to variables that are related to hospital performance and utilization. The research utilized is a descriptive and quantitative study that will seek to determine how TennCare implementation has affected performance and utilization of these hospitals. The analytic research employs the interrupted time series design, which is intended for a study where several observations are made prior to, and after introduction of the independent variable.[91]

The independent variable is TennCare reimbursement and the dependent variables are average daily census, discharges/admissions and measures of economic performance profit) of disproportionate-share hospitals. The unit of analysis will be the year. Economic performance of the hospitals is determined by analyzing profit of these hospitals within the ten year period under study. Effects on average daily census and admissions/discharges are also analyzed.

Population Size: All disproportionate-share hospitals in Tennessee are included in the study. Hospitals that are not classified as disproportionate share are included to serve as controls.

Financial Performance: The focus is on financial performance i.e. profit of Tennessee Hospitals both before and after implementation of TennCare i.e through the years (1989 through 1993) prior to and after (1994 through 1998) implementation of the independent variable. Hospitals that do not treat a disproportionate share of low income individuals are regarded as control hospitals. The analysis is to be carried out with data gotten from Joint Annual Report of Hospitals. The annual reports were obtained from Office of Health Statistics and Information. This office is under the auspices of Tennessee Department of Health (TDH). Tennessee Department of Health obtains yearly data[92] from all hospitals in the state through surveys. As such the study utilizes secondary data sources, but it is important to note that the Tennessee Department of Health's yearly surveys have 100% response rate. This is because the hospitals are mandated to provide such information to the state. Profit of disproportionate share hospitals will be compared with that of control hospitals. William Cleverly's determinant[93] of hospital performance will be utilized. According to Cleverly, the main determinants of hospital performance would include: Outputs, expenses as a measure of Outputs, total productivity rates and input resources prices, net revenue and net profits. But for the purposes of this analysis, only profit will be utilized as a measure of financial performance for all hospitals.

Admissions and Average Daily Census: Data pertaining to these two criteria will also be obtained from Tennessee's Office of Health Statistics and Information.

Regression analysis would be utilized for admissions/discharges, average daily census and profit. Statistical analysis will determine if TennCare implementation had a statistically significant impact on the above mentioned indicators.

As mentioned previously a hospital will be assumed to serve a disproportionate amount of low income individuals if it satisfies HCFA disproportionate hospital classification.

Since as mentioned previously, TennCare is structured so that managed care companies take over management of former Medicaid patients that are now insured under managed care plan, it is possible that the infrastructure that provided indigent care in the east would be undermined especially since the reimbursement rates of TennCare are so row. On the other hand, TennCare extended coverage to many indigent patients who were previously uninsured, thereby possibly reducing the indigent care burden on disproportionate share hospitals. It is also feasible that the managed care plans would redirect patients among hospitals thus providing disproportionate-share hospitals with either more or fewer admissions.

The previous discussion would lead towards the development of three hypotheses to address the research question of whether disproportionate share hospitals fare better under TennCare than previously. The hypotheses are stated as follow:

Hypothesis One: Implementation of TennCare resulted in an increase in average daily census for disproportionate share hospitals.

Null Hypothesis One: Implementation of TennCare resulted in same or decreased average daily census for disproportionate share hospitals.

Hypothesis Two: TennCare implementation resulted in increased hospital discharges/admissions.

Null Hypothesis Two: TennCare implementation resulted in the same or decreased hospital admissions.

Hypothesis Three: The implementation of TennCare resulted in increased profit of disproportionate share hospitals.

Null Hypothesis Three: The implementation of TennCare resulted in the same or decreased profit of disproportionate share hospitals.

Need For the Study

Fundamental changes have occurred in United States health market, since origination of intense national and state wide debates concerning health care reforms. These market changes have manifested themselves especially at state level, where the bulk of health care reforms are taking place. Despite the fact that the public's elected representatives have largely not accepted broad governmental system reform, the nature and pace of health care market changes is still being affected by the public sector.[94] Accordingly, in some communities or states, this is manifested in aggressive governmental activities, while other communities are transformed by the market into a "hands-off" policy environment.[95] But each locale's unique political, fiscal and cultural histories as well as the balance of power among interest groups reflect the divergence in the different approaches.

During the past one or two decades, the majority of the states have at least toyed with the idea of some form of initiatives to reform their health care delivery systems so as to control costs and expand coverage and access to health care. These initiatives by the states were also fueled by federal policy, especially possible Medicare cuts and Medicaid block grants. A variety of estimates indicate that current health care expenditures could be cut at least in half by eliminating unnecessary, inappropriate and avoidable utilization.[96] These extreme estimates might have encouraged states to move towards managed health care plans, since these plans generally utilize a primary gatekeeper to keep down unnecessary utilization.

All levels of government utilize five types of public policy tools in influencing the way that health care is financed and provided. These tools include regulation, taxation, funding of public programs, purchase of services, as well as provision and collection of information. These tools have been wielded in addressing a broad range of policy issues, which include the two key issues of the past two decades, namely spiraling costs of health care and decreasing access to health care.[97] It follows then that the use of these tools by policy makers, would be dependent on the outcomes of "experimental initiatives" tried or carried out by some of the states. If these trials indicate favorable results, then there is the possibility that other state or even federal reform initiatives might attempt to follow the route taken by these states. This will invariably affect health care public policy in the country.

The word "policy" is usually used to describe the most important choices made in organized or private life. Public policy has been described in different ways by different authors. According to Peters, policy is the sum total of all government activities that have an influence on the lives of citizens.[98] Ripley and Franklin[99] define policy and its process as follows: "policy is what the government says and does about perceived problems." For the purpose of this research, Dye's definition of public policy will be utilized.[100] Accordingly public policy is defined as "whatever governments choose to do or not to do." Thus implementation of TennCare was chosen by Tennessee government and therefore would be considered as public policy.

Literature search, of both published and unpublished materials related to the book's topic indicate that there has been no study or article focusing specifically on effects of TennCare on hospitals that serve a disproportionate share of low income individuals. There have been studies pertaining to:

TennCare and academic medical centers: The lesson from Tennessee[101] and Trends in total hospital financial performance under Medicare prospective payment system.[102] Dissertation topics have also focused on related aspects of this research. Such dissertation topics include: The structural response and performance of general hospitals in a managed care environment;[103] Effects of Medicare reimbursement on home health care.[104] Medicaid and Medicare: An implementation study of the Tennessee Primary care network.[105] These studies while being related are quite different from this particular analysis in that the focus on this study will be on TennCare specifically and on all hospitals in Tennessee that serve disproportionate share patients. The study that would be considered most similar to this analysis is Darrell J. Gaskin's work pertaining to the impact of HMO penetration on the use of hospitals that serve minority communities.[106] The study indicated that growth in HMO penetration was associated with a reduction in patient volumes for minority hospitals. It also indicated that HMO penetration was correlated with an increase in outpatient visits for non-minority hospitals.

This book will take the idea further in that instead of focusing on just minority hospitals, a broader approach will be utilized and all disproportionate share hospitals will be studied in Tennessee under TennCare. It is important to study the effects of this reform plan on disproportionate-share hospitals especially since such hospitals are the major source of indigent care, and there is a dearth of information pertaining to effects of TennCare on them. The findings would be compared with that of non-disproportionate share hospitals in the same state. TennCare implementation could erode the patient base and financial performance of disproportionate share hospitals, in that more patients are not covered and as such can pay for medical services, and thus be more inclined to seek medical relief for their ailments. But since these patients now have insurance, they might choose to go to other hospitals, or the managed care organizations may redirect these patients to lower cost hospitals.

The research findings can be important to policy makers, health care administrators as well as public administrators at the federal and especially the state level. At the policy level it is important to note the speed with which the program was implemented despite opposition from different constituent groups, which could offer possible insights into policy implementation strategies. The fact that Tennessee prior to implementation of TennCare was a state with minimal managed care experience offers a sort of natural experiment. The dramatic change that occurred as part of the shift from minimal to maximum managed care involvement and provision of health care for uninsured individuals would provide a good backdrop for further policy studies. Implementation of TennCare Tennessee has given other states something to emulate in their ongoing efforts at Medicaid reforms. In fact, many states have implemented Medicaid reform plans that utilize managed care, and this is mostly due to the general belief is that current health care expenditures could at least be cut in half by eliminating unnecessary, inappropriate and avoidable utilization.[107] This belief is probably the basis for state reforms that lean toward managed health care plans, since these plans generally utilize a primary gatekeeper to keep down unnecessary utilization.[108] But few states have implemented changes as dramatic as the TennCare program. It is thus important to study this innovative plan that was designed to curtail increasing health care costs while at the same time providing more coverage for individuals. Understanding the impact of TennCare on disproportionate share hospitals is important because Tennessee has a significant number of uninsured individuals despite the expansion of coverage accomplished by the reform. Thus, safety net providers, such as disproportionate share hospitals continue to be a vital component of Tennessee's health care system. As more states move their Medicaid population into managed care, the Tennessee experience could provide valuable insights for policy makers.

Chapter 2
Review of Related Literature

The literature review of this study encompasses varied areas relating to TennCare. Chapter one covers some of the background literature leading up to the evolution of TennCare. This chapter continues where chapter one left off, especially with regards to specifics of the program. It also provides the major reasoning behind implementation of the program, covered services and delivery plan. This chapter reviews some of the policy issues surrounding TennCare implementation. The chapter presents some of the problems in the delivery plan as well as the implementation model of TennCare. In order to appreciate the effects of TennCare on disproportionate-share hospitals it is necessary to provide an extensive literature review and background with regards to the reform plan.

TennCare

The TennCare proposal was announced in April of 1993 by Governor McWherter. The proposal called for repeal of the state's hospital tax and extension of health insurance coverage to most Tennesseans that do not have access to employer or government sponsored health insurance. The proposal also called for mandatory enrollment of the entire existing Medicaid population as well as new eligibles into capitated managed care networks. The General Assembly of the state, enacted a two page stature that gave the governor the okay to seek a federal waiver and subsequently implement the program by an Executive Fiat.[109] McWherter, who had been a supporter of Bill Clinton's presidential candidacy, petitioned the White House to grant the waiver, while state Medicaid officials worked hard to prepare for TennCare's implementation. The approval was finally granted in November 1993 by Department of Health and Human Services.[110]

TennCare is basically a Medicaid program operating under a waiver from the federal Department of Health and Human Services and Health Care Financing Administration (HCFA) to the state of Tennessee.[111] The Federal law that affects Medicaid contains clauses that permit "waiving" of exact compliance with all of its details so that a state can basically operate the program with a lot more flexibility than the original law specifies.[112] The main reasons for trying to operate the Medicaid program differently is the opportunity to control overall costs, to cover populations that are considered ineligible under Medicaid, and to support necessary services that are not covered by traditional medical insurance programs. The uninsured and the uninsurable under the reform plan would be added to the number of those already served through Medicaid, and these individuals would then have the opportunity of choosing one of several managed care organizations (MCO). The number of available providers was designed to be dependent on this choice, thus some individuals might have to change their doctors, and likewise some providers might also lose some of their previous Medicaid patients. All these factors were considered in the development of TennCare.

Not only is TennCare supposed to address Tennessee's health care problems, in the best case scenario it should provide an important opportunity to demonstrate potential solutions to national health care concerns. This is because Tennessee's health coverage problems seem to parallel that of the nation as a whole. United States spends more on health care than any other industrialized nation, although proportionately fewer citizens have insured access to the health care system. Just as in Tennessee, national health care costs are on the increase. In 1980 America spent $250 billion on health care costs, and in 1992 more than $800 billion was spent, by 1998 the amount spent on health care had increased to $1.2 trillion.[113] Annual expenditure for 1980 health care was approximately $1000 per person, while the 1992 expenditure was about $3000 per person.[114] Without significant changes to the health care system, national expenditures will exceed $2 trillion by the year 2000 and cost per person will near $5700 per person. Although health care costs have continued to rise, access to health care system has continued to decline, mostly as a result of lack of health care insurance.[115]

Since 1980 the number of people in the population below the age of 65 without health insurance has increased by more than 25%, and this number would have been higher if the federal government had not increased coverage under Medicaid.[116]

TennCare utilizes many of the cost containment measures being considered by the federal government, including, managed care, using the market to set the best price for specified benefit packages (in this case Tennessee would set the capitation rate) and aggregating a large purchasing group to maximize market power.[117] TennCare should also ensure quality of care due to the fact that the different health plans would have to compete for enrollment on the basis of cost and quality of care.

According to McWherter, TennCare was designed to accomplish the following goals:[118]

a) Increase access to health care within a context of overall market-based /global budgetary limits.

TennCare would represent a very large aggregate purchasing pool. As a result it should command significant market power, which should make it possible to provide and ensure quality care coupled with strict quality control at the best possible price. Due to market based pricing, providers would also be forced to adopt cost controls and improve health care management. TennCare would also utilize managed care and capitated payment system. The reform plan would rely on utilization of primary care providers and accountable health plans to check rising costs and over utilization, while at the same time encouraging preventative care.

b) Encourage preventative care

The use of incentives would be employed by TennCare to ensure access to and use of preventive care. Though some enrollees would pay deductibles and co-payments for non preventive care, a wide array of preventive services would be provided at no additional charges (beyond the insurance premium paid by some enrollees). The state would measure the success of this emphasis on preventative care by outcome testing using a variety of health indicators.

c) Improve quality of care

TennCare's structure makes use of significant financial incentives for health plans to maintain quality of care. Accountable health plans would compete for enrollment based on quality of care. The plans that have the best service would get the highest enrollment from all the communities in the state. The program would be administered on a community wide basis. The state would withhold a portion of the capitated payments of the providers pending regular quality reviews by auditors.

d) Incorporate use of charity care funds

Hospitals, doctors and other providers had always provided a substantial amount of charity care to the uninsured. TennCare would reduce overall program expenditures by making use of some of the charity care being provided and thus working that contribution into the program's budget. This would allow Tennessee, to capture market based expenditures already in the system instead of imposing special taxes on the providers. This makes the program suitable for maintaining current level of resources available to the state for provision of health care. The program would also ensure against financial windfalls to providers that otherwise would have resulted from covering patients previously treated on a charity basis.

e) Provide enrollees incentives for appropriate utilization

TennCare would use an innovative cost sharing system that would provide incentives to enrollees on an ability to pay basis. This should discourage unnecessary utilization of unnecessary care. These cost sharing mechanisms would include deductibles, coinsurance payments and co-payments for services excluding preventative care that are charged on a graduated basis to enrollees (other than mandatory Medicaid eligibles) that have income of more than 100% of federal poverty level. This would be done so that payments would not exceed ability to pay, while keeping necessary care affordable and simultaneously providing the appropriate level of incentive to discourage unnecessary utilization.

f) Remove disincentives for AFDC (Aid to family with dependent children) recipients to work

Under the old system, an AFDC recipient who loses eligibility for AFDC after accepting employment will lose eligibility for Medicaid as well, irrespective of whether the new employer will offer health insurance benefits with the new job or not. This acts as a disincentive to work. TennCare negates this disincentive by providing coverage to all uninsured Tennesseans including AFDC recipients that get jobs without health insurance coverage.

g) Encourage coverage of presently uninsured employees and their families, as well as the uninsurables

Under TennCare the uninsured population would have access to health care as long as the uninsured individual does not have access to employer sponsored health insurance either directly or through a family member. Prices would not be tied to employer groups, but would allow the uninsured to buy coverage through employers at the employer's option.

h) Provide continuity of coverage despite changes in status

TennCare would provide continuous access to health care for all eligible enrollees by combining both the Medicaid population and the uninsured populations. This should relieve most of the constant need to reevaluate eligibility for TennCare. Instead enrollees would be able to maintain their enrollment in TennCare, while co-insurance payments and other cost sharing methods are adjusted according to changes in the enrollees' ability to pay. It was hoped that the global budgeting approach, managed care, cost sharing systems, capitated payments. and the preventative care components, under TennCare, would generate sufficient savings that would make it possible for extension of health care benefits to the uninsured population with minimal increase in overall level of health expenditures.

Eligibility Criteria

Three groups of Tennesseans would be covered under the program. Members of these three groups lack conventional health care insurance and they are as follows:

Medicaid enrollees (about a million in number) including both AFDC and chronically disabled group; the uninsurable citizens who cannot get insurance due to present or prior medical conditions;

Individuals who were not eligible for employer or government-sponsored (e.g. Medicare) health plan as of March 1 1993;[19]

Individuals that could be eligible for another insurance program, (even of limited scope) but choose not to enroll in them would not be eligible for TennCare. An initial enrollment cap of 1.775 million was proposed and this cap included individuals from the three groups mentioned previously, thus providing health insurance coverage for about 98% of all Tennesseans.[120]

The federal government seemed skeptical about the state's ability to provide adequate coverage for a larger number of citizens without major increases in expenditures. So it capped total enrollment at 1.4 million and mandated that the state of Tennessee should procure evidence that each chartered managed care organization (MCO)[121] had a physician panel sufficient to provide coverage. The state was also required to document adequacies of MCO's quality assurance and information management plans as well as conduct broad patient satisfaction surveys.[122]

Covered Services

The provision of all approved services to beneficiaries was the responsibility of MCOs.[123] These services would include a wide range of inpatient and outpatient services e.g. preventive care for beneficiaries up to age 21 years, comprehensive hospital and physician services, laboratory and x-ray, home health care medications, medical equipment and supplies, and emergency ambulance support. These services were covered on a limited basis under Medicaid.[124] Limited inpatient psychiatric care for chronically mentally ill would also be provided as well as limited inpatient substance abuse care and outpatient mental health services. TennCare's plan did not include extended long-term mental health care. Medicare premiums, deductibles and selected other services, amounting to almost $1 billion per year would not be covered under TennCare but would be reimbursed as under the old Medicaid program.[125] Generally the program was slated to provide for a broader range of services than that previously covered by Medicaid.

The Delivery Plan

TennCare delivery scheme for ifs enrollees is based on chartering MCOs,[126] that compete to enroll eligible citizens. The MCOs will be responsible for providing the whole spectrum of services covered by TennCare for each individual plan member. Health care will be directly provided by these health plans or they will subcontract with other providers that can provide these services. The TennCare initiative currently had about 12 MCOs in the program.[127] These MCOs were established on either a statewide or regional basis. The state for purposes of TennCare is divided into 12 regions. These regions were established under the community health agency act to coordinate services to the indigent.[128] An MCO can provide service in one or more regions and each beneficiary will have to choose one of the MCOs that operate in their particular region of the state. Preexisting conditions will not be used as an excuse to deny enrollment, and beneficiaries will have the option of changing MCOs annually.[129]

Out of 9 health maintenance organizations (HMOs)[130] and 29 preferred provider organizations (PPOs)[131] that provide services in Tennessee, only Blue Cross /Blue Shield and the Tennessee Primary Care Network[132] eventually became MCOs. The other 10 MCOs that provide health services were established especially for TennCare. The MCOs are supposed to operate as either PPO or

HMOs. Of the 12 chartered MCOs, 4 are PPOs while 8 are HMOs, though the majority of TennCare patients are enrolled in a PPO plan.

This is because the MCO that serves almost 50 % of the enrollees (Blue cross /Blue Shield) is a PPO.[133] HMOs in Tennessee are mandated to maintain a sizable capital reserve, but PPOs are not, thereby increasing risk to providers.[134]

Cost Sharing

The deductibles, premiums, and co-payments of TennCare services are graduated based on income, with maximum deductibles set at $250 for a single individual and $500 for a family per year. Those individuals in mandated Medicaid eligibility groups and those with incomes under the federal poverty level are not required to cost share.[135]

Budgeting and Capitation Systems

MCOs under TennCare are paid based on a capitation system. This system is based on a state wide global TennCare budget, that was originally proposed by the state of Tennessee for the year 1994.This budget included $2.27 billion federal, $383 million state, $255 million in federal and health care funds for other care programs and $50 million for local government spending. About $230 million was expected in premiums, co-payments and deductibles from about 658,000 enrollees that have incomes above the poverty level while $595 million was estimated for the charity care that would remain under TennCare.[136] Under this budget the 6.75 % tax on providers would be eliminated. Due to elimination of the provider tax, the state's hospital industry expressed some degree of initial support for the planned budget. TennCare had an initial proposed global budget of $2.9 billion, but after months of extended negotiations with HCFA an initial annual budget of $2,192,950,800 was established for TennCare. An annual capitation rate of $1,641 was established per person based on this budget. The capitation rate was further discounted to $1,214 by the anticipated local government contributions, continuing charity care, and average beneficiary co-payments. This was then further adjusted based on gender, age, severity of illness, (for example $607 per year was set aside for children aged between 1 to 13 years, and for the blind and disabled it was as high as $3,789). Payment of providers by the MCOs was based on negotiated rates. Over a 5 year demonstration period the overall budget was expected to increase 5% each year after the base year (1994) at a rate equal to the state's economy growth rate.[137] The state requested that federal contributions to TennCare be increased at the same rate as the program's global budget but not to exceed per capita cost rate of growth of 8.3%. TennCare targeted a $2.8 billion reduction of the annual health care expenditures by FY 1997-98 with a cumulative $7.2 billion saving by the end of the 5 year demonstration period, thereby enabling significant cost savings by both the state and the federal government. The initial TennCare per capita rate would be almost the same as that for Medicaid if mean out of pocket expenses and inflammatory costs up to the year 1994 were added. Therefore, the state anticipated that TennCare's rate would be comparable to both reported Medicaid and state employee per capita rates, though TennCare would be providing a much broader range of services than Medicaid.[138]

The dependability and validity of these comparisons are questionable. It has not yet been shown with a degree of certainty that the plan actually enables significant cost reductions for both the state and federal governments. Some journal articles seem to imply that the plan appears to have placed undue financial stress on hospitals or health care centers that serve TennCare patients)[139]Despite that, there are varied factors that make it difficult to actually estimate or dispute the presumed cost savings. For instance, TennCare population might be sicklier, than commercial HMO's enrollees or state employee groups. This is because TennCare is not supposed to practice discriminatory selection based on medical history. Thus all the enrollees that are eligible would automatically be included with disregard for their medical history. This would tend to increase costs over comparisons groups.[140]Another point worth noting is that the state might have underestimated prior costs of Medicaid by assuming that all beneficiaries had received a full year of coverage, whereas the actual average period covered for individual Medicaid recipient was approximately 8.7 months.[141] This misrepresentation would present a lower estimated cost than the actual annual cost. The start up costs for the MCOs were also not taken into consideration. The inclusion of 5% charity contribution, though lower than Medicaid's, also builds cost shifting into TennCare while at the same time there is no guarantee of full health coverage of all Tennesseans.[142] Lastly, although the $1,641 gross capitation rate might be close to other benchmarks, the MCOs were paid a 25% discounted rate, thereby giving them an incentive to obtain 25% discount on services, over current rates. This discount rate would be considerably higher than the cost savings or discount on services of other MCOs.[143] Thus the actual health status of TennCare beneficiaries might not have been correctly portrayed by current Medicaid group because the majority of eligible citizens enroll in Medicaid only when they become ill. On the other hand it would be conceivable that TennCare beneficiaries enroll in the program even when healthy. Therefore it would be likely that the healthy eligible citizens' enrollment might actually reduce the overall cost and severity level of the population that are eligible for TennCare. For example children and their parents from low income single parent families (which tend to resemble the profile of newly covered beneficiaries) constituted 72% of Medicaid beneficiaries, though they cost only about 32% of Medicaid expenses.[144]

Participants Involved in TennCare Policy and Implementation

Public policy as mentioned previously can generally be defined according to Peters,[145] as "The sum total of government activities that have an influence on the lives of citizens." TennCare fits within the context of this description. The program can be seen as a culmination of government activities that have an influence on the lives of Tennessee (TN) citizens, especially on TennCare beneficiaries. Ripley and Franklin[146] on the other hand define policy and its processes as follows, "Policy is what the government says and does about perceived problems." Within this description can be superimposed the processes of TennCare. The program can be considered the end product of TN state government activities that were directed towards solving the issues of lack of health care insurance and escalating health care costs. It follows then, that the word "policy" is usually used to describe the most important choices made in organized or private life. One could then conclude that policy making is how the government decides what will be done about perceived problems.

Cahn[147] (1995) indicates that policy making is a process of interaction among governmental and non-governmental policy actors, whereas policy is the outcome of that interaction. Policy actors are described as both formal and informal individuals and groups, who seek to affect the creation and implementation of these public solutions.[148] Policies can be described within two different but important senses: how they are made and how they can be made better.[149] As such it is necessary to study policy making and implementation so as to "learn" how to make and implement better policies.

According to Stella Theodoulou,[150] the common stages of policy development include the following:

a) *Problem Recognition and Issue Identification*: This is the stage where the attention of policy makers are drawn to a problem that could require governmental action; legitimate problems can then develop into issues.

b) *Agenda Setting*: This involves recognizing the problem or issue as a serious matter.

c) *Policy Formulation*: At this stage different proposals are developed for dealing with the issue.

d) *Policy Adoption*: This involves efforts that are made to obtain enough support for a proposed solution, to make it to the government's stated policy.

e) *Policy Implementation*: At this point the policy mandate is achieved through public programs and the federal or state bureaucracy, and usually with citizen, state and local government cooperation.

f) *Policy Analysis and Evaluation*: This particular process involves examining outcomes of implemented policy and determination of the success of the policy. The author mentions that the above process should be viewed as an ongoing cycle that should involve the monitoring of policy, so as to see how well it is serving the intent of its implementation.

The policy stages outlined above could be utilized in tracing the development of TennCare. The state of Tennessee recognized that there was a problem regarding escalating health care costs and high number of uninsured individuals. As such the problem was set on the agenda, with ensuring proposals developed for dealing with the issues. The most viable proposal was then adopted and consequently implemented. The various articles and studies on TennCare would constitute the analysis and evaluation stage of the program. The analysis can take various forms, e.g, looking at the outcome of the program as a whole or instead taking sections of the program and analyzing it for educational or policy purposes.

Public policies can not execute themselves and as such, effective implementation is needed before decisions of policy makers can be carried out. Usually the people that determine public policies are not the ones to carry them out. Instead there are various participants that take part in both policy making and implementation of policy. The majority of policies require an intricate and sometimes complex set of positive actions on the part of a lot of people, so as to be implemented.[151] Stella Theodoulou indicates that implementation starts after the decision has been made to undertake a specific course of action, and ends when the goals sought by the policy have been achieved within reasonable cost estimates.[152] The author also describes implementation as the directed change that follows a policy adoption.[153] Eugene Bardach on the other hand, views the implementation procedure as a two step process that involves: The assembling of different components necessary to produce a specific programmatic outcome; and the playing out, of a number of loosely interrelated games where these components are delivered or withheld from the program assembly process based on particular or specific terms.[154] Sabatier and Mazmanian see implementation as comprising of statutory structures, problem tractability as well as nonstatutory forces. As such there are varied components in the implementation process. These components affect the achievement of policy objectives and would include social, economic, technological conditions and the target groups that are involved.[155] So according to Sabatier and Mazmanian, the success of a policy being implemented depends on factors such as:

Tractability of the problem including;
1) Availability of valid technical theory and technology.
2) Diversity of Target group Behavior.
3) Percentage of the target group relative to the general population.
4) The Magnitude of behavioral change needed.
Ability of Statute to Structure Implementation involving;
1) Clear and consistent objectives.
2) Incorporation of sufficient causal theory.
3) Financial resources.
4) Hierarchical integration with and among implementing institutions.
5) The decision guidelines of implementing agencies.
6) Hiring of implementing official.

7) Formal access by outsiders.
Non statutory Variables Affecting Implementation such as;
1) Socioeconomic conditions and technology.
2) Attention of the media to the problem.
3) Public support.
4) Resources and attitudes of the different constituency groups.
5) Executive support.
6) Leadership skill and commitment of implementing officials.

Some of the above mentioned components and their subsequent effects on TennCare implementation are incorporated within this chapter.

Former Governor Ned McWherter, was a major participant in the TennCare process. In early 1993, the then Tennessee Governor, stated that he would make Tennessee the first state in the nation to "withdraw from Medicaid." This he managed to do, by obtaining a federal waiver, under Section 1115 of the Social security Act. This waiver made it possible for launching of a managed care program that affected the state's whole health care delivery system.[156]

Roles of Different Constituents to TennCare Implementation

Successful implementation of any policy requires (to some extent) conducive attitude on the part of constituent groups. But in the case of TennCare, different constituents or interest groups in Tennessee had almost no say or input in implementation of the program. One of the Governor's strategy for speedy implementation of the program was intentional exclusion of possible detractors from the implementation process. Thus health care provider interest groups that were against TennCare had insufficient time to detract from implementation of TennCare.[157]

The Tennessee Hospital Association (THA) and Tennessee Medical Association (TMA) were among the critical interest groups that opposed the TennCare proposal.[158] The THA believed that TennCare should be run as a managed care program with full risk being borne by insurance carriers. On a different vein, the organization did not think that it was realistically possible even under TennCare to insure significantly more citizens without a resultant state health care funding increase.[159] Since it was not apparent that state funding increase was imminent, members of the THA were apprehensive about methods the state would utilize in undercutting possible cost increases that would occur with more enrollment. It was difficult too for THA to accept the proposal that health care resources would be used by Medicaid patients at the rate predicted by state employees. It was inconceivable to them that there would be enough enrolled physicians to provide the needed services nor was it conceivable that sufficient funds would be generated from enrollees to cover the costs of the program. It was quite possible that with unlimited enrollment, there would be a concurrent increase in cost shifting to other insurers. There could also be an increase in the amount of charity care provided.[160] THA wanted the state of Tennessee to provide sufficient proof as to actuarial soundness of TennCare and adequacy of the capitation rate when pitted against the amount and variety of services to be provided.[161]

The TMA had much stronger objections. Their main objection stemmed from the development of the plan without input from healthcare providers. The organization also objected to the idea of physicians' increased risk for malpractice suits while practicing under the managed care requirements. The increasing enrollment without enough funding (i.e the inadequate capitation rate) was also another source of contention for the organization. Tennessee Medical Association members did not appreciate the fact that the financial status of TennCare and the MCOs were kept secret. Under TennCare, PPOs would not be placed at risk by their contracts instead the financial risk would be transferred from the state to the providers.[162] The organization was vehemently opposed to the requirement by Blue cross/Blue shield that physicians should participate in TennCare if they wished to participate in other plans like the Tennessee Provider Network (TPN). The TPN was a more lucrative plan, that served state employees and other customers. In fact the TMA's opposition was so strong that they filed suit against the State of Tennessee to block TennCare implementation, but their suit was dismissed by both Tennessee state Court of Appeals and the Chancery Court on grounds that the TMA did not have a case since the physicians were paid by MCOs and not by the state.

The National Association of Community Health Center (which represents 700 federally funded health centers) filed a suit to block implementation of TennCare and they also filed a suit against the United States Department of Health and Human services for not enforcing TennCare waiver conditions.[5][163] According to Mirvis et al. the major concerns of the Association were as follows:

i) There was too little implementation time to allow proper development of needed delivery systems and administrative structures. This could result in confusion and hamper the proper implementation of the program.[164]

ii) There was not enough protection against adverse selection. Since the program was supposed to cut costs by enforcing community rating on prices, setting standard benefits and guaranteeing access to every one regardless of health condition, it was most probable that insurers would try to discourage sicker patients from enrolling in their plans. They could also limit access to high quality care and specialists thus causing patients who needed such care to try and enroll in other plans.

iii) The association members were apprehensive that adequate information would not be provided to beneficiaries in the enrollment process. Because of the short implementation time it would be very difficult for adequate information to be provided for the insured. Information that the insured would need included lists of available network doctors for different specialties and their different regions or areas of practice within the state.

iv) The level of payment was at least 25% less than the costs of providing care. In fact according to the state medical association, TennCare payments are about 40% of the cost of delivered services while the Medicaid program had been paying about 50 % of the cost of services rendered.

v) Finally, there was not sufficient physician participation and cooperation. This was due to TennCare's low payment rates and tedious guidelines for participation. This caused a lot of doctors and health insurers to avoid participation in the program. For example when TPN (Tennessee Provider Network)[165] mandated that it's participating doctors would have to take TennCare patients, about half of the network's 6,400 doctors dropped out because they did not want to be involved with TennCare. But by August 1994 most of the doctors had rejoined the net work because of a substantial drop off in the number of their patients. A lot of the large managed care networks in Tennessee such as Aetna Health Plan, Provident Life and Accident and Pru Care decided not to join TennCare.[166]

The National Association of Community Health Centers in their suit appeared to be concerned among other issues, that the state had not met most of its condition for waiver approval by HCFA.[167] Initial media reports of the proposed reform plan had been very glowing, but these media reports increasingly turned negative in the face of negative reaction from the interest groups mentioned above.

Despite all the initial opposition TennCare was implemented very rapidly, it came into effect on January 1, 1994, just 43 days after final HCFA approval and less than 9 months after announcement of the program.

One important issue to consider is the ability of the state of Tennessee to implement TennCare relatively quickly, on schedule without any major structural or programmatic changes from the original plan. A lot of factors were responsible for making this possible. Governor McWherter skillfully engineered the plan with just a small group of his advisors and with hardly any public debate nor input from providers and insurers. The Governor announced the plan around the end of annual legislative session. The element of surprise was crucial in approval of the plan in broad conceptual form from state legislature. To keep this element of surprise intact, the details of the plan were published while the legislature was out of session.[168]

The program was to be implemented by January of 1994, which would present the returning legislature with an already established program that would be more difficult to restructure. This made it possible to avoid a probable political debate that could have delayed, reshaped or blocked the program development as is usually the case at national level. The primary design of TennCare as an extensive expansion of the state's Medicaid program, rather than as a fundamentally new program helped aid speedy implementation. So there was a sort of incremental approach to the implementation of this program. Paul Schulman describes the strategy of incrementalism as one of continual policy readjustments in search of marginally redefined policy goals. As such, long term plans are discarded in favor of short term political implementation[169]. This strategy was inherent in implementing TennCare as an expansion program in lieu of being implemented as a radically new program. Since the legislature did not have the time to explore the proposed TennCare legislation in detail due to the timing of the proposal, members of the legislature either had to accept or reject the proposal. Since the proposal seemed very promising at first glance, it was almost given that state legislature would be irrevocably committed to TennCare's implementation at reconvening of the legislature for the 1994 January session. Then the probability of undue and irresistible pressure from interest groups would not have much effect on their earlier authorization of the program. So it was strategically necessary to try and implement TennCare reform by 1 January, 1994, regardless of whether or not it was ready to be implemented.[170]

Governor McWherter focused on health care financing and delivery systems reforms rather than on the probable limiting impacts on insurance or malpractice systems. This approach quite likely reduced complexity of the plan and breadth of possible opposition. The state and the Governor also had great confidence throughout the process of the application for approval of the waiver, that it would be granted. Accordingly, despite notification that HCFA approvals might be delayed, the state still went ahead and mailed TennCare enrollment documents to eligible beneficiaries on its pre-established timetable.[171] All these factors when compiled together helped make it possible for TennCare to be implemented as quickly as it was.

How Implementation of the Program Defined Content of the Policy

The broad policy goals of TennCare's implementation were the reduction in health care costs and increased coverage. The implemented program could be evaluated on those criteria to determine if the reform was able to define the content of the policy during implementation. To do that it is necessary to elaborate on achievements and problems that surfaced after implementation and thus determine if the content of the policy was actually defined or not.

Achievements of TennCare

TennCare enrollment reached 1.27 million at its peak period, and this is equivalent to more than 25% of the approximately 5 million citizens in the state. The enrollment figure includes 850,000 former Medicaid recipients and 419,000 formerly uninsured persons. Under TennCare health insurance of all Tennesseans under the age of 65 years increased from 89% in 1993 to 95% in 1994 (the highest of all the states). Blue cross/Blue Shield had about 49% of the recipient enrollment, while the state's seven smallest groups had only a combined enrollment of 10%.[172]

The state also claimed to have met the financial goals of the program, indicating that TennCare saved an estimated $1.6 billion within the first 18 months of the program in state and federal funds based on conventional Medicaid expenditure growth rate. At the same time the program enrolled more than 400,000 new people. There was also increased funding by the state for the seriously mentally sick, as well as for MCOs that had a lot of high cost patients.[173] There was likewise increased health care funding for youths, as well as for sole community hospitals and primary care providers that serve a very large number of TennCare recipients.[174]

It is possible to concede that the state did a good job in implementing TennCare, because it was able to implement fairly quickly and on schedule the major tenements of the reform plan. Although there were some initial start up problems, one could argue that the problems did not require major structural or programmatic changes for the initial plan. That in itself could be considered a major achievement.

Problems of TennCare

Despite the claims of success that can be attributed to TennCare, it is also necessary to elaborate on the problems of implementation. Due to the rapidity with which TennCare was implemented, it was difficult for both the state and the 10 new managed care groups to organize adequate delivery and information systems. Therefore it was tough for the already existing plans to develop new policies and procedures. This resulted in confusion during the initial enrollment period, and as a result the state initiated a second enrollment period in December 1993.[175]

There were significant backlogs in processing enrollment applications due to the rapid implementation. The state as mentioned previously was unable to send premium payment booklets to about 80,000 monthly premium paying enrollees resulting in great a deal of revenue loss. In fact during the early months of implementation there was so much confusion that the state returned premium payments to some enrollees that had already paid their premiums. This was because they did not have adequate accounting systems to account for both the enrollees that had paid and those that had not. The state also provided wrong and incomplete enrollment data to MCOs as a result of their inadequate data management systems.

Some MCOs included some shady deals in their enrollment practices, e.g they offered inducements such as secured credit cards and life insurance to enrollees, they directly enrolled non-eligible individuals such as prison inmates and they directed potential clients with costly and life threatening diseases to other MCOs.[176] There was also problem of inexperience on the part of MCOs as mentioned previously. Out of the 12 MCOs that were initially operating at the onset of TennCare, only one of them had previous experience with managed care for Medicaid populations.

Some of TennCare premiums were not collected from enrollees and there was more rapid enrollment of beneficiaries than was projected. This contributed to a $99 million deficit reported by TennCare bureau in January 1995. There is also a possibility that the amount of deficit would be greater[177] if outstanding bills, were taken into account. Tennessee also owed HCFA over $100 million in matching funds received during FY 1993-94. HCFA maintained that the state, in it's request for federal matching funds, inappropriately included certified public expenditures. State officials maintain that the $99 million deficit is relatively small when compared to what the deficit would have been if the Tennessee Medicaid system had still been in effect.

As a result of some the above mentioned problems, coverage of chronically mentally ill patients was delayed. The state stopped enrolling uninsured citizens with incomes over the Medicaid eligibility limits as of January 1995.

One of TennCare's policy objectives was to save money by cutting costs for the state but it seems that to the extent that Tennessee's government costs were lowered, health care providers or the federal taxpayers simply picked up the tab. A lot of the MCOs seemed to be having financial problems. Some of these MCOs reported third quarter (1994) deficits that were more than $2 million. Blue Cross/Blue Shield of Tennessee (the largest of TennCare MCO reported a first year loss of $8.8 million).[178] It is important to address the financial performance of health care facilities or providers because if most of the plans' providers were to go bankrupt it would be difficult to provide health care to insured individuals. The unpaid bills of collapsed MCOs could not be covered by the state thereby shifting further fiscal responsibility to providers.

Hospitals also seemed to be having problems under TennCare. In the first 6 months of 1994 the average hospital received 44 cents from MCOs, for each dollar spent on a TennCare patient, resulting in an annual loss of $47 million. These hospitals had 2 options in order to cover these losses. They had the option of either reducing overall expenses by 9 % or raising charges to other carriers by 17% i.e. increasing cost shifting. The hospitals were also receiving 28% less reimbursement under TennCare than under Medicaid. State officials also notified hospitals that payments amounting to about $217 million total in 1994 were going to be deferred. This payment was supposed to be made out to hospitals for medical education costs and to essential and sole community providers for uncompensated care incurred. It was supposed to cover care provided to non enrolled but eligible citizens. As a result of all these funding problems some of the hospitals, especially public hospitals planned on reducing graduate medical educational programs, clinical services, and number of their employees. Due to a $42 million shortfall out of $208 million TennCare total budgeted funding, the state's largest public facility (Regional Medical Center in Memphis) stopped giving care to uninsured individuals from outside its home county. The Center also curtailed some specialized programs like the AIDS program, reduced residency positions and were planning to reduce its total workforce by 20%.[179]

There were also problems of patient and physician dissatisfaction. Only about 49% of former Medicaid patients surveyed considered their care under TennCare to be as good as or better than under Medicaid.[180] The state approved Consumer Advocacy Program in 1994 claimed that there had been up to 2,720 complaints regarding TennCare. About 17% of the complaints were related to enrollee problems, 35% were about individual MCO functions and 46% were complaints concerning the state's TennCare office. The enrollees also complained about processing, application delays and changes in MCOs by the state. Some of the MCOs that were enrolled in the program complained about insufficient number of specialists, benefit misrepresentation and disagreements over the necessity of some medical procedures.[181] More than 90% of the physicians surveyed believed that the rigid drug guidelines of managed care plans prevented them from effectively treating their patients.[182]

The state also utilized discretionary funds to offset fiscal effects of TennCare's implementation. This was done by making payments to essential providers as well as underwriting much of the care that was delivered out of plan.[183] There were still thousands of uninsured Tennesseans and the particular market forces utilized by TennCare would make it very difficult for the uninsured to obtain charity care in the private sector.[184] TennCare has made it possible for termination of subsidies, effective from 1996 for major public hospitals and health centers in Memphis and Nashville.[185] Thus far it was still undetermined whether disproportionate share health care centers are faring favorably or unfavorably under this reform plan, and that is the basis of the study.

It could be argued that implementation of TennCare achieved to some limited extent the major outlines of the policy goals. By the end of 1994, TennCare had achieved an enrollment of 1.2 million (300,000 formerly uninsured Tennesseans) and 94.6% of the residents of Tennessee had some form of health care coverage, more than that for any state so far.[186] Tennessee's budget crisis was also under control. This is as a result of TennCare's capping of rate of future growth of Medicaid expenditures. The projected revenue discrepancy, $99 million in a total budget of $1 billion, was manageable and did not require as Medicaid had threatened to do, a major realignment of the state's budget.[187]

Summary

As far as state level health care reforms go, TennCare seems to be amongst the most ambitious and comprehensive, due to among other things, the size and scope of it's delivery systems and the speed with which it was implemented.[188] Ned McWherter employed a main strategy of managed care which was new to Tennessee, to bring about reform for the state. Before TennCare, only about 5.9% of the total population were enrolled in managed care systems, and of these only about 2.7% of Medicaid patients were enrolled in managed care system. The Medicaid system that the state of Tennessee had, required individuals to be at the low end of the poverty threshold with almost no other assets before they could be eligible for Medicaid benefits. Unlike Medicaid, TennCare will make it possible for a working poor person that makes between 100% and 200% of the federal poverty level[189] to afford health care premiums and deductibles. This is because these premiums and deductibles are based on a sliding scale. Therefore as a person makes more money, they would gradually assume a greater portion of their insurance payment, and at above 200% poverty they will assume full deductible payment and premiums. Almost all of Medicaid recipients and about 25% of the total state population are included in the program.

TennCare was implemented with the following broad policy goals in mind:

a) Expansion of services to all those that needed medical services without the addition of new taxes;

b) Insuring that every Tennessean that is not insured would be covered by the program;

c) Saving Tennesseans about $6.5 billion in health costs by the year 2000 and,

d) Saving the federal government $1.5 billion by the year 2000.[190]

One of the above mentioned goals of the program i.e. that of cost reduction while expanding coverage is based on two financial and health delivery innovations, namely managed care and global budgeting . According to data from Medicaid managed care systems, the managed care strategy has the ability to help reduce utilization and costs.[191] Hurley et al evaluated 25 Medicaid managed care programs and out of the 25 programs evaluated, 19 reported cost reductions, two showed cost increases and the rest had no change in expenses.[192] This indicates that there is the possibility that TennCare (which utilizes managed care) if managed properly could provide advantages for the state on a long term basis. The possibility for this needs to be determined.

Zwanziger and Averbach , reported that non-Medicaid populations had higher medical expenses under fee for service plans than under TennCare.[193] This argument would seem to support the state's view that managed care plans will reduce costs.

Another impressive thing to note about TennCare is the speed of implementation by Tennessee state government. This speedy implementation might have been aided by designing the plan as an extensive expansion of the state's Medicaid program rather than as a fundamentally new program. Also the fact that the reform was directed on delivery systems and health care financing, limited the impact on insurance or malpractice systems and helped keep the plan simple while reducing amount of possible opposition. This strategy possibly helped implement the plan faster. The fact that the state went ahead and mailed TennCare enrollment forms to eligible beneficiaries based on its' pre-established timetable while awaiting the delayed approval from the HCFA also helped speed matters up, though had the state not gotten the needed approval it would have been in a bind for doing that. Its' assumption that it would get the needed approval worked out for the state in this instance.

Organized physician and hospital groups still continue to oppose TennCare as a result of growing financial losses, while the shaky financial and fiscal viability of the MCOs seem to foretell of more losses to providers as well as threaten the disruption of care to patients if no action is taken to improve matters.

The state currently is under the Governorship of Bredesen, who is the second governor of Tennessee since McWherter left office. Governor Bredesen has instituted several broad and sweeping changes to TennCare. These current changes will be discussed further in Chapter 5.

It is safe to say that TennCare has reversed the main paradox of American health care, which involves continuous increases in health care spending followed by a proportional decrease in the number of insured Americans. Its methodology of controlling inflation while expanding coverage has so far provoked wide skepticism. Cutting through a broad ideological spectrum, a number of analyzes seem to agree that the program is little more than an extension of the old "creative financing" technique.[194] Kinder analyses of TennCare seem to regard it as a "miracle" with an underlying implication that it cannot be replicated by others.[195] Therefore it is necessary to evaluate and analyze TennCare so as to determine how beneficial it could be for future health care reform plans.

Chapter 3
Methodology

This chapter describes the methodology used in the study of effects of TennCare reimbursement on disproportionate share hospitals. As such the chapter is comprised of the research design, the research questions and postulated hypotheses. Operationalization of the hypotheses is also described followed by discussion of the population in the study. The later part of this chapter focuses on the procedures for data collection.

Research Design

This study examines the effects of TennCare reimbursement on disproportionate share hospitals. An interrupted time series design was utilized for this study. A time series design is usually used when there are multiple observations over time. The observations can be on the same units e.g. when particular hospitals are repeatedly observed, or they can be on different but similar units, e.g when yearly grade point average of each graduating class in a particular university are displayed over a series of years. In the later case there would be different students in each graduating class each year.[196] In the former case the same hospitals are observed for different years. The interrupted time series involves making several observations prior to introduction of the independent variable and several observations after the fact. In this type of analysis it is required that the researcher should know the specific point in the series when a treatment occurred i.e, when the independent variable was introduced. This is because the intent of the analysis is to infer whether or not the independent variable had any impact on the dependent variables.[197] If the independent variable caused some impact on the dependent variable, it is expected that observations after the treatment would be statistically different from those before it. That means that the series would show signs of an 'interruption" at an expected point in time.[198] O'Sullivan and Rassell state that the interrupted time series design helps demonstrate that exposure to the independent variable brought about the change(s) in the dependent variable which could not be attributed to long term trends, cycles or seasonal events.[199] Accordingly, a number of observations are made prior to and after introduction of the independent variable. This research design tries to determine if introduction of the independent variable resulted in (1) an abrupt permanent change in the dependent variable; (2) an abrupt temporary change, which lessens and returns to normal level after a while; or (3) a gradual permanent change whereby the initial change either gradually increases or decreases before tapering off.[200]

With the interrupted time series design the independent variable could be introduced by the researcher but it is usually something that has been introduced by some one else or something that occurred naturally. In most cases the introduction of the independent variable has occurred prior to study by the researcher. This is particularly true in the case of studying TennCare. This design was chosen because it appears to be the best suited for purposes of this study. A number of observations (hospital data records for the years before TennCare) were made prior to introduction of the reform program and after introduction of the independent variable. The independent variable in this instance is TennCare. The hospital data provides information that will help determine whether introduction of TennCare resulted in an abrupt or gradual permanent/temporary change in average daily census, discharges/admissions and profit of disproportionate share hospitals. This would be contrasted with the effects on non disproportionate share hospitals. As mentioned previously the non-disproportionate-share hospitals will serve as controls. This is so as to control for effects of seasonal changes and trends.

The research design is diagramed as follows:

$$O_1\ O_2\ O_3\ O_4\ O_5\ X\ O_6\ O_7\ O_8\ O_9\ O_{10},$$

where O_1 represents observations starting from the year 1989, and O_{10} represents observation for the year 1998.

Research Questions and Research Hypotheses

The purpose of this study is to determine the effects of TennCare reimbursement on disproportionate-share hospitals (DSHs). The results of this study will help demonstrate whether or not implementation of TennCare had a positive effect on average daily census, admissions/discharges and profit of disproportionate-share hospitals. Although TennCare is administered as a managed care program with low reimbursement rates for medical treatment of enrolled individuals, it is likely that the covered individuals would tend to more actively seek medical care for medical problems since they do not have to worry about paying for the bulk of medical services rendered. This could contribute to higher patient volume and revenues. Disproportionate share hospitals may not experience as much bad debt because many previously uninsured individuals gained coverage under TennCare. Although the DSHs, would be paid a discounted rate for services, they would at least receive some reimbursement in lieu of no reimbursement at all as was the case in the past when they treated indigent patients that had no means of paying for services rendered. In this case half bread (i.e. about 50%

discounted rate of payment by TennCare for services rendered to enrollees) would be better than nothing as far as their financial bottom line was concerned. This could result in more admissions and possibly better financial performance for these hospitals than before implementation of TennCare. Alternatively, under TennCare, MCOs could avoid contracting with DSHs resulting in decreased admissions and revenues. Also if under TennCare, MCOs reimbursement rates are inadequate to cover costs, net revenues could fall. These ideas led to the formulation of the research question. The research question is expressed as follows: Does implementation of the health care reform plan (TennCare) lead to increase in average daily census, discharges/admissions and profit of disproportionate share hospitals? This research question can actually be broken down to include the following hypotheses.

- *Hypothesis One*: Implementation of TennCare resulted in an increase in average daily census for disproportionate share hospitals.
- *Null Hypothesis One*: Implementation of TennCare resulted in same or decreased average daily census for disproportionate share hospitals.
- *Hypothesis Two*: TennCare implementation resulted in increased hospital discharges/admissions.
- *Null Hypothesis Two*: TennCare implementation resulted in the same or decreased hospital admissions.
- *Hypothesis Three*: The implementation of TennCare resulted in increased profit of disproportionate share hospitals.
- *Null Hypothesis Three*: The implementation of TennCare resulted in the same or decreased profit of disproportionate share hospitals.

The independent variable for all the above hypotheses is the implementation of TennCare. The normal approach in a time-series regression equation is to include 3 created independent variables, which would be utilized to capture the effects of the interruption. These three independent variables include: The dummy variable where 1= the presence of a policy (in this case TennCare) and 0 = the absence of the policy. The counter variable or the linear trend variable where I = the first year of the time series, 2 = second year of the series and so on. The last created independent variable for the time series is the post-policy intervention counter variable where 0=each year prior to TennCare implementation and 1,2,3.. .n is for each year after the policy.[201] The effects of these variables in the analyses will be discussed further in Chapter 4. The dependent variables for the individual hypotheses are as follows:

- *Hypothesis One-* Average Daily Census
- *Hypothesis Two-* Hospital Discharges/Admissions
- *Hypothesis Three-* Hospital profits.

Data

In order to determine the effects of TennCare reimbursement on disproportionate share hospitals, secondary data obtained from Tennessee Department of
Health (TDH), Office of Health Statistics and Information were utilized. The
data base or Joint Annual Report of Hospitals, from the Office of Health Statistics (OHS) included the names and addresses of all hospitals in the state of Tennessee. The Joint Annual Report of Hospitals also contained information pertaining to utilization, occupancy and financial performance of all the hospitals
that are contained within the database. Thus the data revealed utilization (admis-
sions/discharges and average daily census) and financial performance (profit) of
the hospitals in Tennessee, for years prior to and after TennCare implementation
i.e 1989 through 1998. The data for all hospitals in the state of Tennessee were
utilized for the study. The state has an average of 160 hospitals, but the number
varied from year to year due to the fact that some hospitals merged or closed and
some new ones opened within the period of study.

Data pertaining to hospital utilization were available as hard copies from
OHS, while data pertaining to profit was available on floppy disks. The hospital
utilization data (for all the hospitals for the 10 years) was entered manually onto
the database. Since there was the possibility of making mistakes in the process
of manual entry of data, it was necessary to randomly spot check the entries to
make sure that the data was entered correctly. The rest of the data set i.e those
containing information pertaining to financial performance of the hospitals were
then transferred from the floppy disk to the researchers computer hard drive.
The two data sets were then merged via use of state identifier tax codes or numbers for each hospital. The tax identifier for each hospital was assigned to both
the data on the floppy disk and the data set that was originally on hard copy. The
resulting database was converted to SPSS format.[202]

The data in the SPSS format was then utilized in calculating the descriptive
statistics on the demographic, utilization and financial data. The results were
then analyzed statistically to determine statistically significant differences and
co-relationship using SPSS. The results of the statistical analyses of the data are
presented in chapter four.

Population

The population for this study is all the hospitals in Tennessee. As such data from
all the hospitals in the different counties in the state were utilized. The lists of
the hospitals in the state, from years 1989 through 1998 was utilized. The lists
were cross-checked to note the hospitals that had changed their names or the
hospitals that were no longer in existence. For the hospitals that were no longer
in existence or that did not report their performance and utilization rates for particular years, the computer recorded the years that such hospitals did not have
their reports in, as missing data. There was no sampling in this case since all the
hospitals were analyzed.

The disproportionate share hospitals were a subset of the population. They were also analyzed separately, and then compared with the performance of non-disproportionate share hospitals during the study interval.

Hospitals

The data reported in the Joint Annual Report of Hospitals, allowed for comparison of hospital characteristics with the utilization and financial performance results. The hospital characteristics included information pertaining to utilization, admissions/discharges and HCFA classification as disproportionate or non-disproportionate share hospital. These demographics were obtained from Office of Health Statistics and Health Care Information Agency (HCIA) which prints annual Profiles of United States hospitals using data gotten from annual Health Care Financing Administration (HCFA) reports. Prior to using the data from HCFA and OHS, it was necessary to determine if the data available was suitable for the purposes of this research. As such, it was necessary to determine what constituted the population and the strategy utilized by the above mentioned agencies in their initial collection of the data.[203] The response rate was also considered. It was also necessary to determine when and how the data were collected and how the data was coded and edited. For purposes of this research, the operational definitions of measures that were utilized by the agency initially collecting the data, had to be considered too.[204]

The above criteria had to be considered so as to make sure that the population represented the population of interest and that the data collection strategy was sufficient to provide a true population estimate. In the case of this research, the Department of Health (DOH) regularly surveys all the hospitals in TN. Surveys are sent each year to all the hospitals on the state listing of hospitals. The hospitals are mandated to provide their yearly reports to the office, so response rate was about 100%. The data were collected yearly via cost report sheets turned in by the individual hospitals. These data were then coded and edited by the statistical/data analyst for the office. The operational definitions of measures are explained in Operationalization of variables.

Data gotten from HCFA generally denoted the location/teaching status of the hospitals and type of care provided by the hospitals. The data also denoted the hospitals that were classified as disproportionate share hospitals. The classification by HCFA should be considered valid since HCFA is the federal agency that makes the determination of whether or not a hospital is disproportionate share or not. Thus HCFA's classification of the hospitals were matched to the hospital lists generated by the DOH. Therefore, hospitals that were classified as disproportionate share were identified using the state identifier code or tax identification number and the letter D. This identification was necessary to differentiate between these hospitals and the other non disproportionate share hospitals for purposes of statistical analysis and testing of hypotheses. Statistical analyses of the data involved the utilization of multiple regression models, to test the hypothesis. The depth of the statistical analysis utilized for this research would be presented in Chapter 4.

According to the Tennessee Department[205] of health the following should be noted when interpreting the data:

A. Financial Data:

1) The instructions required that all questions pertaining to finance be completed using the same accounting method required by HCFA for the Medicare cost reports, but it is possible that some hospitals might have utilized different accounting system. So there is the possibility that the data might not be strictly comparable.

2) Financial data were omitted for specific hospitals if the facility was open less than six months.

3) Some facilities were able to provide only financial totals with no detailed breakdowns.

4) The data that were included in total calculations, were strictly those for facilities that reported both numerator and denominator data. For those hospitals that did not provide sufficient information for the calculations, that particular variable was left blank.

B. Utilization Data: Totals for the computed variables were based only on hospitals reporting all necessary components for the computations, otherwise the space for the variable was left blank.

C. Reporting Period: Though the hospitals were asked to report data for the calendar year, some facilities reported the data for their fiscal year.

Operationalization of Variables

This study examined the independent variable-TennCare reform plan, and the dependent variables-average daily census, discharges/ admissions and profit. The time series analyses also utilized the three created independent variables in analyzing the effects of TennCare on disproportionate-share hospitals.

The reform plan TennCare is operationalized as the plan that took effect in 1994 that transferred Medicaid patients and uninsured individuals to managed care plans. It can be considered a nominal variable. It should be noted that TennCare did evolve over the years and HCFA changed the percentage of poor points required for some hospitals to qualify for DSH payments. But for the purposes of the study, any hospital that has ever been classified as a disproportionate share hospital was treated as one.

The three dependent variables are ratio type variables. Utilization or average daily census is operationalized as the number listed in average daily census of each individual hospital. The average daily census is defined as the average number of patients in a facility on any day of the reporting calendar year. Rate of utilization could also be characterized by total inpatient days which is the number of adult and pediatric days of care rendered during the whole reporting period. An inpatient day of care or a patient day or a census day (can also be classified by some federal hospitals as an occupied day) is a period of service between the census-taking hours on two successive calendar days. The day of discharge is included, only when the patient was admitted the same day. Patient discharge/admission is operationalized as the number of both adult and pediatric patients (excluding newborns) admitted to the facility during the reporting period.

Financial performance is operationalized as the total financial well being of the hospital, and it takes into consideration revenues generated in the process of running the hospital. Profit[206] was utilized as a measure of financial performance is operationalized as the excess of revenue over expenses.

Disproportionate share hospitals (DSHs) are categorized or identified by HCFA as those hospitals that have an appreciable Medicaid patient base. Since these hospitals serve a disproportionate number of indigent patients, payment rates for the hospitals are increased or adjusted (DSH adjustments). This is done to counter the disadvantaged position of these hospitals that treat a larger than usual number of indigent or Medicaid patients. In-order to be classified as a DSH, the hospital should have a disproportionate patient percentage (DPP) of 15 percent.[207] This percentage is derived by adding the sum of two fractions, namely, the Medicare/Supplemental Security Income fraction and the Medicaid fraction.[208] After the Omnibus Budget Reconciliation Act (OBRA) of 1993[209] was passed, only the hospitals that fit specific criteria of at least 1% Medicaid inpatient utilization rate could receive disproportionate share payments.

Validity and Reliability of Using the Interrupted Time Series Analysis

Whenever a researcher is undertaking a quasi experimental research, there is the possibility of bias due to the very nature of this kind of research. Quasi experimental design usually lack some of the characteristics of experiments and some of the control afforded with them. Accordingly, a researcher might need to rely on a naturally occurring independent variable or base comparisons on groups over which the researcher has no control. Thus quasi experimental designs reduce the researcher's ability to judge the impact of an independent variable.[210] Therefore, such a design can never prove that one variable causes another. But having a model and showing that the variables are statistically related, that the independent variable occurs before the dependent variable and that other possible causal independent variables have been ruled out makes a more solid case for a causal relationship.[211]

Therefore in evaluating a program to see if it has the hoped for results, it is necessary to show evidence that the independent variable brought about changes in the dependent variable. In a time series design, information is collected on a dependent variable at several time points before and after implemented policy, so as to assess the impact of the policy. Interrupted time series means that it is expected that the policy innovation being studied (over time) have changed or interrupted trends in the dependent variable.[212]In order to eliminate threats to internal validity it is necessary to control for factors other than the policy change that might affect the dependent variable.[213] A study or research can be said to be internally valid if a researcher is confident that the independent variable of interest caused change in the dependent variable.

External validity on the other hand refers to the issue of a researcher being able to generalize the findings of a study beyond the specific cases involved. Operational validity focuses on whether the methods utilized for measuring a variable make it possible to actually measure the criteria that needs to be measured. Internal validity questions if a researcher's protocol enables the researcher to claim that the cause of a change in a dependent variable has been identified.[214] As such when one is undertaking a study it is prudent to identify possible threats to the validity of the research and try to minimize threats to validity of the research.

The interrupted time series is suited for this research because it controls for the effects of maturation since observations were taken prior to and after implementation of TennCare. This type of research design also controls for the effects of statistical regression since it allows for assessment of the pre and post effect trend.[215] The main threat to internal validity with this type of research is the effect of history. This effect is usually due to other events occurring at about the same time as the introduction of the independent variable, but this is controlled in this research by checking state records to make sure other major events did not occur within that period. Three independent variables were utilized as part of the regression equation to counter the effects of history and other unmeasured effects that might occur. These variables are the time counter variable, the dummy variable and the post policy variable. The time counter for year takes account of history and other unmeasured effects that may occur over time. It is a term for change in intercept and it is coded 1 ,2,3,--n, for the number of years of the study.[216] Where 1 is for the first year (1989) in the time series; 2 for the second year and so on till 10 for the last year (1998). This is a linear trend variable that takes into account long term trends in economy and hospital growth. This coefficient thus indicates the average yearly level of increase in the dependent variables, when computed for the whole 10 year period.[217]

Another variable called the dummy variable was created, where 1= the presence of the policy, and 0= the absence of the policy. Thus all years prior to 1994 would be coded 0 and all years from 1994 and after would be coded 1. Therefore the dummy variable is like a difference of means score, it provides the difference in mean of the dependent variables before and after TennCare implementation.[218]

The third variable is the post-policy intervention counter variable which allows the researcher to measure the changes that occurred after introduction of the policy. This is coded 0 for each year before the policy was adopted and 1, 2, 3, ...n for each year after policy adoption.[219] Thus the years 1989 through 1993 will each be coded 0 but 1994 = 1, 1995 = 2 .... 1998 will be coded 5. These variables are the time series variables and will be utilized in the time series analyses. The regression equation for the time series analyses is as follows:

$$Y = a + b_d x_d + b_t x_t + b_p x_p + e$$

where:

x_d = The dummy variable before and after TennCare implementation

x_t = Counter variable from 1989 to 1998

x_p = Post-policy counter variable, equal to 0 before TennCare adoption and 1 through 5 afterwards.[220]

Selection effects as a threat to validity was checked by making sure that there was no major change in the population (hospitals) being measured. As such it was important to cross check the number and names and tax identities of the hospitals in TN to make sure that changes in number per year were very slight. The changes in number per year was limited to a maximum of 3 or 4 per year, if any at all. Experimental mortality was not a serious problem since the total missing data were about 10 for the 10 years under study.

Threats to external validity were minimized, especially since interaction between selection and treatment were minimized by the fact that all the hospitals were surveyed and all the hospitals were subjected to the TennCare climate. The fact that the independent variable TennCare was introduced all at once and at a clearly identifiable time hopefully should make the effects easier to identify.

Cook and Campbell[221] indicate that possible construct validity concerns for time series involve two scenarios or criteria. These criteria would include;

i) A situation where the same respondents (hospitals in this case) are repeatedly measured, whereby the repeated measurements would impinge on the respondents' reaction to the independent variable.

ii) Another scenario that might impinge construct validity would be a situation where by respondents were cognizant of implementation time of the treatment (introduction of the independent variable). This might subsequently bias their behavior or reaction to the independent variable, but Cook and Campbell also indicated that these two criteria are usually not met and in the case of TennCare research, the two criteria were not met so it is assumed that there is no problem with construct validity.

Welch and Comer[222] on the other hand, indicate that in time series it is necessary to be aware of two main factors that could affect the validity of the findings. One of the factors is trend. The time series procedure should consider the effects of long term trends on data analysis. Another factor is seasonality or cycles in the pattern of economic growth, which could affect the results of the analysis.[223] Economic growth might fluctuate on a regular cycle, with a few years of "boom" followed by a few years of slow economy. This sort of cyclical pattern should be considered in determining the impact of a particular policy. If for instance, the policy intervention occurred at the bottom of the cycle, it could appear to have positive effects when in actuality it did not. On the other hand if it occurred at the top of the cycle, it might appear to have negative effects.[224] In order to control for the effects of trends, history and seasonality the dummy, time counter and post policy variables as mentioned previously, were utilized in the regression analyses.

Special Problems of Time Series

Multicollinearity. Usually time series equations have small number of cases. For example this study where N =10. This makes it likely that a multicollinearity problem will develop.[225] Multicollinearity, describes a situation whereby the independent variables are correlated. This is a problem because with the different independent variables being correlated it becomes very difficult to disentangle their effects. The collinearity statistics thus measures the level of correlation between independent variables. The variance inflation factor (VIF) is used to measure the level of collinearity. If the VIF is less than 10 then there is no collinearity problem, but if it is greater than 10 then there is a collinearity problem.

Auto-correlation. This is used to describe the correlation of error terms.[226] The DurbinWatson (D-W) statistic determines the level of Auto-correlation. It determines auto-correlation between the series of results gotten over the 10 year period of study for that particular variable. The D-W statistic can vary from 0 to 4. The closer it is to 2, then the less likely it is that there is a problem of Auto-correlation.[227] For purposes of this study a value that is around 2 will indicate no correlation, which would be considered good, since the regression model assumes no auto correlation. But on the other hand if there is significant Auto-correlation in the results, then corrective action will have to be taken. This involves transformations of the variables used in the equation and estimation of the equation.[228] The above mentioned problems of time series analysis will be addressed in Chapter 4, when analyzing the data.

Chapter 4
Data Analyses

This chapter contains the statistical analyses and interpretations of the data collected in order to determine the effects of TennCare reimbursement on disproportionate share hospitals. The first three chapters have described in some detail factors relating to the concept of health care system in the United States, literature relating to TennCare, data collection, and the analytic methodology utilized for this study.

The first section of this chapter describes the population and statistical analyses results using descriptive statistical techniques. This chapter takes into consideration the effects of demographics on the results. An overview of the effects of the reimbursement schema is also presented. The second part of this chapter examines the data results in relation to the hypotheses postulated. It also relates general perceptions and attitudes about TennCare to the findings. Conclusions drawn from analyses of the data are presented.

Hospital Characteristics

One important characteristic of this research is that all the hospitals within the state of Tennessee were analyzed. As such, averages of 160 hospitals per year were analyzed for the years 1989 through 1998. Since the state obtained utilization and financial data from the hospitals, response rate was 100%. There were cases where some hospitals failed to turn in their raw utilization data form on time (for that particular year), which meant that their data for that particular year would be considered invalid or missing for the purposes of this research. Some of the hospitals also had instances where specific information for a particular variable would not be included and as such that particular variable would be considered a missing variable. Despite this the response rate should still be considered 100% since all the hospitals (for the most part) provided the information required by the state, except as mentioned before in the rare instances that the information was not provided on time or was not applicable.

In order to address the hypotheses, it was necessary to differentiate between non-disproportionate share and disproportionate share hospitals. The analyses focused on both non-disproportionate and disproportionate share hospitals, as admissions (operationalized as discharges/admissions) and financial performance of the hospitals (operationalized as profit).

Since all hospitals in the state of Tennessee were included in the study, it was assumed (barring any data collection errors) that data gotten for these analyses are truly indicative of characteristics of hospitals for the period 1989 through 1998. The table 1 below shows the frequencies for HCFA classification of all the hospitals analyzed within the 10 year period. The frequency tables were included as part of the data, so as to provide a breakdown of the number of hospitals that were considered disproportionate share hospitals.

Table 1. Frequencies for HCFA Classification for the Years 1989 Through 1998

Years	Frequency or Total	Percent	DSH	Non-DSH
1989	161	10	89	72
1990	162	10.1	89	73
1991	163	10.1	89	74
1992	159	9.9	86	73
1993	159	9.9	85	74
1994	158	9.8	85	73
1995	154	9.6	82	72
1996	162	110.1	83	79
1997	167	10.4	83	84
1998	164	10.2	83	81
Total	1609	100	854	755

Data Analyses

It is important to know that the data analyses for this study were carried out with a true population data, instead of sample data. As such it is necessary to remember that most statistical tests utilized in demonstrating causality are usually carried out on sample data. According to O'Sullivan and Rassell[229] a test of statistical significance is a type of inferential statistic or procedure. Inferential statistics make it possible for a researcher to infer population characteristics from sample data. Inferential statistics are therefore used to estimate parameters.[230] Parameters can be considered population characteristics. Usually researchers utilize random samples in estimating the values of population parameters. Since population data was utilized for this study, it is necessary to bear in mind that although some statistical analyses were carried out on the results from the data, the fact that samples were not utilized presents a unique characteristic. This should be considered when dealing with or interpreting the results of the statistical analyses. As such the data analyses for the most part consisted of regression analysis, which can be utilized for real population statistics.

The hospitals were grouped into two, that is disproportionate share and non-disproportionate share hospitals. The yearly median of each of the three dependent variables for all the hospitals were then plotted against the years, 1989 through 1998. This was done for both the disproportionate and non-disproportionate share hospitals. The median instead of the mean was utilized because the median is not as sensitive as the mean to possible extreme values which could result from error in data entry, although the means were included in the tables of descriptives. O'Sullivan and Rassell[231] indicate that the mean is usually the preferred measure of central tendency, if the distribution is unimodal and symmetrical or nearly so. But if the distribution has a few extreme values, either high or low, then the mean would be distorted or the distribution considered skewed. In such cases the median should be used instead of the mean.[232]

The mean and median for average daily census for both disproportionate share and non-disproportionate share hospitals prior to and after implementation of TennCare are shown on table 2. The standard deviations are also included, and the same is done for all the tables that are part of the data analyses. Standard deviations show the measures of dispersion or variation within the distribution. Thus, smaller values for standard deviation indicate more uniformity while larger values suggest more variation. The range (highest to lowest value) also gives an idea of how variable the data are, and as such is included for all the tabulated data. It should be noted that the standard deviation and the range are utilized in inferential statistics (which deals with samples), but they can also be used in measuring variability in population statistics. The range and standard deviation are useful population parameters which describe variability in the distributions. They are equally as important as the means and the medians in descriptive statistics. The data analyses are broken down into four parts or sections. The first part deals with analysis of data to determine if the null hypothesis regarding average daily census will be accepted or rejected. It involves analysis of median average daily census to see if TennCare implementation brought about an increase in patient utilization. The second part deals with the analysis of data to determine if the null hypothesis regarding profit will be accepted. It involves analysis of financial performance data to determine if TennCare implementation brought about better financial performance (i.e. will DSHs experience increased profit under TennCare). The third part determines if hypothesis three (i.e. DSHs will experience an increase in admissions/discharges under TennCare) holds true, and it therefore deals with analysis of hospital admissions. The fourth part or section concludes on the data analyses.

Descriptives

Table 2 shows that there is considerable difference between the median and the mean of average median daily census of both DSHs and non-DSHs, and as mentioned before this would imply that there are extreme values that skewed the distribution, otherwise the means would be closer in values to the medians. Prior to implementation of TennCare, the average median of the disproportionate share hospitals on average median daily census was 30 more than that for the non-disproportionate share hospitals. But the average median daily census for disproportionate share hospitals decreased by 12 after TennCare implementation, and that for non disproportionate share hospitals decreased by six.

Average Median Daily Census

Table 2. Average Median daily Census by HCFA CLASS. before and after TennCare

	TennCare	HCFA CLASS		Statistic
Avg. Census	Before	Non-DSHs	Mean	70.5063
			Median	32
			Standard Deviation	102.2545
			Minimum	0
			Maximum	581
		DSHs	Mean	112.3880
			Median	62
			Standard Deviation	127.1685
			Minimum	1
			Maximum	517
	After	Non-DSHs	Mean	57.0493
			Median	26
			Standard Deviation	79.1329
			Minimum	
			Maximum	447
		DSHs	Mean	99.4282
			Median	50
			Standard Deviation	112.6028
			Minimum	3
			Maximum	471

Figure 1: Graph of average median daily census plotted against years for DSHs and Non-DSHs

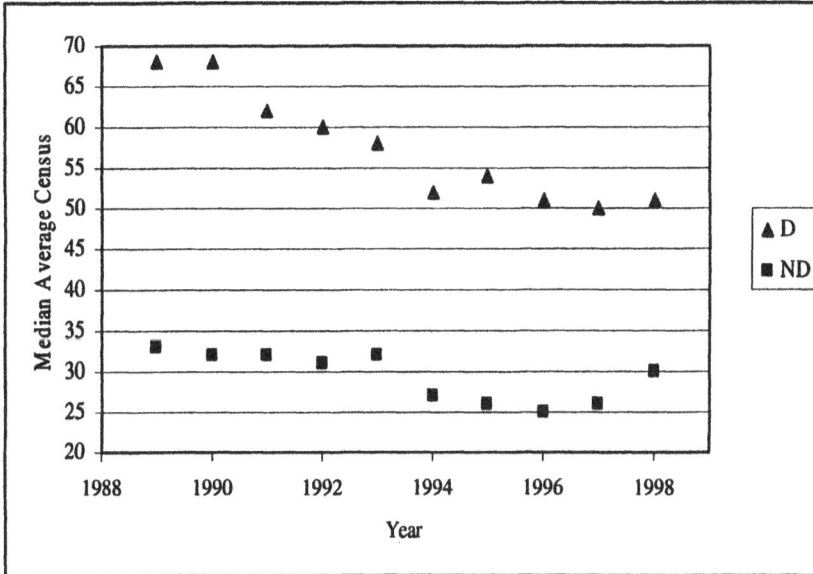

Conversely after TennCare implementation the disproportionate share hospitals had an average median daily census that was 24 more than that for nondisproportionate share hospitals. Thus it would appear that average median daily census of both nondisproportionate and disproportionate share hospitals decreased after TennCare implementation.

When the average median daily census is plotted against years for disproportionate share hospitals and non-disproportionate-share hospitals the graph in figure 1 is produced. The graph shows a downward trend in average median daily census for disproportionate share hospitals prior to TennCare implementation and a decrease in linear downward trend after TennCare implementation. The graph in figure 1, also allows for comparison of the effects of TennCare on both DSHs and non-DSHs simultaneously.

When linear regression analysis was done for year against average median daily census for DSHs, with the three created independent variables, the results shown in table 3 were realized.

Table 3. Regression Analysis for Average Median daily Census for DSHs

Model	R square	R Square Change	Durbin Watson
1	.979	.979	2.837

Model	Unstandardized coefficients		Collinearity Statistic
	B Value		VIF
1 Constant	73.100		
Dummyvar	-3.900		4.250
Counterv	-3.100		8.250
Postplv	2.000		6.500

a. Predictors: (Constant), Postp, Dummyvar, Counterv   b. Dependent
Variable: Dispavdc

Table 3 shows that the R square value is .979. This shows that in using the
model to describe the changes in the data, the model accounts for 98 percent of
the variability in average median daily census over the ten year period. Thus the
R square value of .979 shows that there is a strong linear association between
changes in average median daily census for DSH and TennCare implementation.
The remaining two percent of the model is due to unmeasured effects. It should
be noted that the higher the R square the more confident the model is in terms of
accounting for history and maturation effects.[233] The Durbin-Watson test checks
to see if there is auto-correlation in the series over the 10 year period for the
particular dependent variable. Auto-correlation, is a common characteristic of
time-series data. Auto-correlation describes the nonrandom relationship among a
variable's values at different time periods.[234] Thus the presence of auto-
correlation affects the accuracy of error terms, which biases the model's confidence limits and hypotheses tests.[235] The rule of thumb is that a Durbin-Watson
value of around 2 is desired because that would indicate no significant auto-
correlation, and that would be good because the regression model assumes no
auto-correlation. The Durbin-Watson tests for non-independence because the
regression model assumes independence of the variable over the years of the
study. A Durbin-Watson of between .8 and 1.7 is inconclusive as to the question
of auto-correlation. The Durbin-Watson value of 2.837 indicates that there is no
significant auto-correlation for disproportionate share hospitals' average median
daily census.

The variance inflation factor (VIF) is a measure of collinearity. Multicollinearity measures correlation between independent variables. A VIF value
that is less than 10 indicates that collinearity is not a problem for that particular
regression analysis. Since the VIF of the independent variables are less than 10,
multi collinearity for DSHs average median daily census is not a problem.

The regression coefficients (B) values for average median daily census of
DSHs, show that the trend up to TennCare implementation on average median
daily census was a decrease of 3.1 (counter variable) per year. After TennCare
implementation this trend increased by 2 (post-policy variable) per year. So the

net effect of TennCare implementation is the sum total of post-policy variable effects and counter variable effects. So the net effect of TennCare implementation is a yearly decrease of 1.1 in average median daily census for DSHs.

When considering figure 1, which is the median average daily census plotted against years for non-disproportionate share hospitals and disproportionate-share hospitals, the graph shows a scattered downward trend in average median daily census for non-disproportionate share hospitals prior to and after TennCare implementation.

The regression analyses of average median daily census by year for non-disproportionate share hospitals (with the three created independent variables) produced the results shown in table 4.

Table 4. Regression Analysis for Average Median daily Census for non-DSH

Model	R square	R Square Change	Durbin Watson
1	.749	.749	1.650
Model	Unstandardized coefficients		Collinearity Statistic
	B Value		VIF
1 Constant	33.700		
Dummyvar	-5.300		4.250
Counterv	-.500		8.250
Postplv	1.000		6.500

a. Predictors: (Constant), Postp, Dummyvar, Counterv   b. Dependent Variable: Ndisavdc

The R square value is .749. This shows that in using the model to describe the changes in the data, the model accounts for 75 percent of the variability in average median daily census for non-DSHs over the ten year period. This value measures the strength of the linear trend. Thus the R square value of .749 shows that there is a strong linear association between changes in average median daily census for non-DSH and TennCare implementation. The remaining 25 percent is due to unmeasured effects. Since the Durbin-Watson value is between .8 and 1.7, it is inconclusive as to the question of auto-correlation for average median daily census for non-DSHs.

The VIF of the independent variables are less than 10, so there is no problem of collinearity for non-DSH average median daily census. The regression coefficient or B values[236] show that the trend up to TennCare implementation on average median daily census was a decrease of - .5 per year. After TennCare implementation it increased by 1 per year. The net effect of TennCare implementation on average median daily census for non-DSH is thus an increase of .5 per year. The null hypothesis which states that DSH will experience a decrease or no change in average median daily census is rejected. This is because although there was a net decrease in average median daily census for DSH after TennCare implementation, the downward trend that was visible prior to TennCare appears to be reversing after TennCare implementation.

Profit

Table 5. Profit plotted by HCFA CLASS. before and after TennCare (TC)

	TennCare	HCFA CLASS		Statistic
Profit	Before	Non-DSHs	Mean	714908.82
			Median	24345.000
			Std. Deviation	3370489.3
			Minimum	-3927541
			Maximum	41298765
		DSHs	Mean	2193831.9
			Median	709925.00
			Std. Deviation	4680158.0
			Minimum	-1.5E±07
			Maximum	32926462
	After	Non-DSHs	Mean	1129550.5
			Median	321428.00
			Std. Deviation	5034714.3
			Minimum	-2.4E+07
			Maximum	48988504
		DSHs	Mean	3487358.3
			Median	1234628.5
			Std. Deviation	7737173.0
			Minimum	-3.8E±07
			Maximum	52984066

Table 5 shows that for non-DSHs the median profit appeared to increase by $297,083 after TennCare implementation, while for DSHs median profit appeared to increase by $524,703.5 after TennCare. This means that the rate of increase of profit for both DSHs and non-DSHs prior to TennCare implementation was generally higher than the rate of decrease after TennCare implementation.

When profit is plotted against years for disproportionate-share hospitals and non-disproportionate-share hospitals, the graph in figure 2 is produced.

Figure 2   Profit plotted against years for DSHs and Non-DSHs

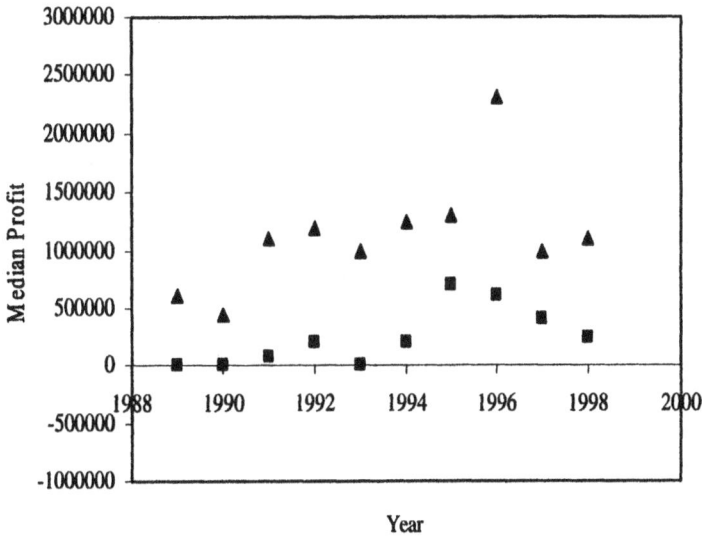

The graph shows no real linear trend in profit for disproportionate share hospitals prior to and after TennCare implementation. But there was a definite positive upward trend in profit for DSHs prior to TennCare implementation. But after TennCare implementation, there was a non-linear but definite negative trend in profit. This accounted for the median profit prior to TennCare being lower than the median profit after TennCare implementation. Thus after TennCare implementation the median profit appeared to be on a downward trend though it is still higher than the median profit prior to TennCare implementation. This is justified by the regression analysis. When regression analysis was plotted for profit by year for DSHs, with the three created independent variables, the results shown in table 6 were produced.

The R square value is .308. This value measures the strength of the linear trend. This shows that in using the model to describe the changes in the data, the model accounts for 31 percent of the variability in median profit for DSH over the ten year period. The remaining 69 percent is due to unmeasured effects. Thus the R square value of .308[237] shows that there is not a strong linear association between changes in average median daily census for DSHs and TennCare implementation. The Durbin-Watson value is around 2, so the regression model has no problem of auto-correlation for median profit.

Table 6. Regression Analysis for Profit for DSHs

Model	R square	R Square Change	Durbin Watson
1	.308	.308	2.197
Model	Unstandardized coeffi-cients		Collinearity Statistic
	B Value		VIF
1 Constant	380046.04		
Dummyvar	253142.58		4.250
Counterv	105193.46		8.250
Postplv	-150512.5		6.500

a. Predictors: (Constant), Postp, Dummyvar, Counterv   b. Dependent Variable: Disprof

The VIF of the independent variables is less than 10 so there is no problem of collinearity for DSHs median profit. The B values show that the trend up to TennCare implementation on median profit was an increase of \$105,193.46 per year. After TennCare implementation it decreased by \$150,512.5 per year. The net effect of TennCare implementation on median profit for DSH is thus a decrease of *\$45,319.4* per year.

When the graph for profit in figure 2 is analyzed, the graph shows no linear trend in profit for non-disproportionate share hospitals prior to TennCare implementation. But the graph shows that there were increases in profit for the first two years after TennCare and then there was a downward linear decrease or trend in profit. The regression analysis was then calculated to produce table 7.

Table 7. Regression Analysis for Profit Non-DSHs

Model	R square	R Square Change	Durbin Watson
1	.566	.566	1.770
Model	Unstandardized coeffi-cients		Collinearity Statistic
	B Value		VIF
1 Constant	24475.2 10		
Dumniyvar	196569.39		4.250
Counterv	8387.030		8.250
Postplv	-13329.54		6.500

a. Predictors: (Constant), Postp, Dummyvar, Counterv   b. Dependent Variable: Ndisprof

The R square value is *.566*. This shows that in using the model to describe the changes in the data, the model accounts for 56 percent of the variability in profit for non-DSHs over the ten year period. The remaining 44 percent is due to unmeasured effects. Since the Durbin-Watson value is between .8 and 1.7 it is not conclusive that there is no auto-correlation for median profit for non-DSHs.

The VIF of the independent variables is less than 10 so there is no problem of collinearity for non-DSHs' median profit. The B values show that the trend up to TennCare implementation on median profit was an increase of $8,387.030 per year. After TennCare, it decreased by $13,329.54 per year. The effect of TennCare implementation on median profit for non-DSHs is thus a decrease of $4,942.51 per year. This is less than the yearly decrease in profit for DSHs after TennCare implementation. Since non-DSH acts as control hospitals for the study, the null hypothesis which states that DSH will experience a decrease or no change in profit after TennCare implementation is accepted.

Discharges and Admissions

Table 8 below shows that the median for discharges/admissions for non-DSHs decreased by 171.5 after TennCare implementation. On the other hand, median discharges/admissions for DSHs increased by 111.5 after TennCare implementation.

Table 8. Discharges and Admissions plotted against HCFA CLASS. before and after TennCare (TC)

	TennCare	HCFA CLASS		Statistic
Discharges/ Admissions	Before	Non-DSHs	Mean	2650.5590
			Median	1637.5
			Std. Deviation	2843.1376
			Minimum	23
			Maximum	14482
		DSHs	Mean	6431.9469
			Median	3727
			Std. Deviation	6813.5882
			Minimum	60
			Maximum	31977
	After	Non-DSHs	Mean	2771.5622
			Median	1466
			Std. Deviation	3609.7222
			Minimum	11
			Maximum	27963
		DSHs	Mean	6730.4248
			Median	3838.5
			Std. Deviation	7079.3480
			Minimum	37
			Maximum	31371

Discharges and Admissions when plotted against years for both non-disproportionate share hospitals and disproportionate share hospitals produced the graph in figure 3. The graph shows a linear downward trend in discharges and admissions for non-disproportionate share hospitals prior to and after TennCare implementation.

Figure 3. Median discharges and admissions plotted against years for DSHs and Non-DSHs

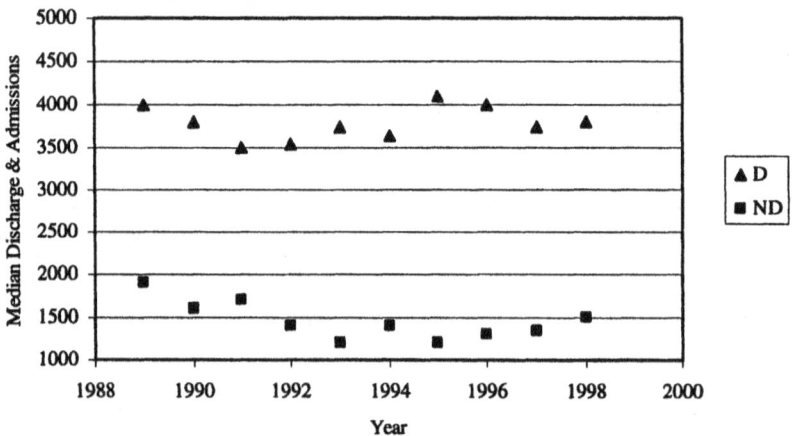

The regression analysis was then calculated to produce table 9 below.

Table 9. Regression Analysis for Discharges and Admissions Non-DSHs

Model	R square	R Square Change	Durbin Watson
1	.746	.746	2.509
Model	Unstandardized coefficients		Collinearity Statistic
	B Value		VIF
1 Constant	2013.100		
Dummyvar	-56.100		4.250
Counterv	-133.9000		8.250
Postplv	179.200		6.500

a. Predictors: (Constant), Postp, Dummyvar, Counterv   b. Dependent Variable: Ndis-adm

The R square value is .746. Since this value measures the strength of the linear trend, it shows that in using the model to describe the changes in the data, the model accounts for 75 percent of the variability in median discharges/admissions for non-DSHs over the ten year period. Since the Durbin-Watson value is 2.5 it is concluded that there is no significant auto-correlation for median discharges/admissions for non-DSHs.

The VIF of the independent variables is less than 10 so there is no problem of collinearity for non-DSHs median discharges/admissions. The B values or regression coefficients show that the trend up to TennCare implementation on median discharge/admissions was a decrease of 133.9 per year. After TennCare implementation it increased by 179.2 per year. The net effect of TennCare implementation on median admissions/discharges for non-DSHs is thus an increase of 45 per year.

The result of regression analysis for discharges/admissions DSHs is displayed below in table 10.

Table 10. Regression Analysis for Discharges and Admissions DSHs

Model	R square	R Square Change	Durbin Watson
1	.288	.288	2.418

Model	Unstandardized coefficients		Collinearity Statistic
	B Value		VIF
I Constant	3905.100		
Dummyvar	325.400		4.250
Counterv	-64.500		8.250
Postplv	59.500		6.500

a. Predictors: (Constant), Postp, Dummyvar, Counterv   b. Dependent Variable: Dis-addis

The R square value is .288. This shows that in using the model to describe the changes in the data, the model accounts for 29 percent of the variability in median discharges/admissions for DSHs over the ten year period. Since the Durbin-Watson value is 2.4 it is concluded that there is no significant autocorrelation for median discharges/admissions for DSHs.

The VIF of the independent variables is less than 10 so there is no problem of collinearity for DSH median discharges/admissions. The regression coefficients or B values show that the trend up to TennCare implementation on median discharge/admissions was a decrease of *64.5* per year. After TennCare implementation it increased by *59.5* per year. The net effect of TennCare implementation on median admissions and discharges for DSH is thus a decrease of *5* per year. The regression analysis thus indicates that median admissions/discharges were on the decrease for DSHs prior to TennCare implementation, but the rate of decrease started reversing after TennCare implementation. The null hypothesis that DSH will experience a decrease or no change in admissions/discharges is rejected because although the regression analysis showed a net decrease, after TennCare implementation, the total effect of TennCare was to increase discharges/admissions. Thus despite the fact that the sum of the post-policy and counter variables were negative, there was a reduction in the downward trend of discharges/admissions after TennCare implementation. The graph in figure 3 shows that on the whole, median discharges and admissions increased for DSHs after TennCare implementation.

Conclusions to Data Analyses

This chapter included the data analyses utilized in testing the three hypotheses of the study. The net effect of TennCare implementation on median profit for non-DSHs is a decrease of $4,942.51 per year. This is less than the yearly decrease in profit for DSHs after TennCare implementation. Since non-DSHs act as control hospitals for the study, the first null hypothesis which states that DSHs will experience a decrease or no change in profit after TennCare implementation is accepted.

The regression coefficients show that the trend up to TennCare implementation on average median daily census was a decrease of 3.1 per year. After TennCare implementation it increased by 2 per year. The net effect of TennCare implementation on average median daily census for DSHs is thus a reduction in the downward trend or decrease of median average daily census. So the second null hypothesis which states that DSHs will experience a decrease or no change in median average daily census is rejected. This is because although there was a net decrease in median average daily census for DSHs after TennCare implementation, the downward trend that was visible prior to TennCare appeared to be reversing after TennCare implementation.

The third null hypothesis that DSH will experience a decrease or no change in admissions/discharges is rejected because although the net effect of TennCare implementation is negative, the regression analysis indicates that median admissions/discharges were on the decrease for DSHs, prior to TennCare implementation, but the rate of decrease started reversing after TennCare implementation. This is indicated by the positive B value or regression coefficient for admission/discharges after TennCare implementation.

Two of the null hypotheses are rejected while one is accepted. The implications of these findings will be discussed in chapter 5.

Chapter 5
Discussion and Conclusions

This book focuses on the policy and rationale behind TennCare implementation. It also incorporated the use of a study to examine the effects of TennCare reimbursement on disproportionate share hospitals. Chapters 1 through 4 focused on literature review and background of the program TennCare, as well as on the methodology utilized and data/statistical analyses for the research. This chapter 5 focuses on summarizing and discussing findings of the data analyzes. This chapter also describes the limitations of the study as well as interprets results of the data analyses within the larger context of public policy implementation. Recommendations and implications for future research and conclusions drawn from the data analysis are also incorporated into this chapter.

The first section focuses on review and discussion of major findings of the data analyses as well as limitations of the study. The second section addresses results derived from the data analyses. It also addresses the public policy significance of the study. This chapter then concludes with implications and recommendations for future research directions.

Summary and Discussion

A time series research design was utilized in determining the effects of TennCare's reimbursement on disproportionate share hospitals. Secondary data spanning ten years was collected from the Tennessee Department of Health, Office of Health Statistics and Information. These data concerned utilization and financial performance of hospitals in the state. Using HCFA classification, the hospitals were then further categorized into disproportionate and non-disproportionate share hospitals. Data for these hospitals were then analyzed for the years prior to and after TennCare implementation. The research sought to answer the question: Did the implementation of TennCare in Tennessee affect utilization and financial performance of disproportionate share hospitals?

The introduction and literature review examined the status of increasing health care costs in USA and specifically in Tennessee and efforts directed by the state in trying to control spiraling health care costs. Thus the first two chapters of the book shed some light as to why it was necessary for the state of

Tennessee to reform its' Medicaid program so as to try and control increasing health care costs and provide more inclusive insurance coverage for its indigent citizens. The reform plan implemented by the state on January 1994 was the independent variable of the study. There were also 3 created independent variables namely the dummy, counter and post-TennCare variables. Average daily census, discharges/admissions and financial performance (profit) were the dependent variables.

The three hypotheses developed for the study are as follows: 1) Hospitals that serve disproportionate number of low income individuals will experience better financial performance (profit) under TennCare than previously. 2) Disproportionate-share hospitals will experience an increase in average daily census under TennCare than previously. 3) Disproportionate-share hospitals will experience an increase in admissions/discharges under TennCare than previously.

The null hypotheses developed for each of the three dependent variables are as follows: 1) Hospitals that serve disproportionate number of low income people or individuals will experience negative or no improvement in financial performance after TennCare implementation. 2) Disproportionate-share hospitals will experience a decrease or no change in average daily census after TennCare implementation. 3) Disproportionate-share hospitals will experience a decrease or no change in admissions/discharges after TennCare implementation.

Two of the three null hypotheses were rejected while one of the null hypotheses was accepted. The first null hypothesis was that implementation of TennCare would result in same or decreased financial performance. This null hypothesis is accepted. This is because the regression analysis showed that the net effect of TennCare implementation on profit of disproportionate-share hospitals through the years spanning 1994 through 1998 was a decrease of $45,319.4 per year. This decrease is significantly more than the yearly decrease in profit for non-disproportionate-share hospitals. When table 5 is considered, then it could be seen that after TennCare implementation, median profit for non-disproportionate-share hospitals increased by $297,083, while that for disproportionate-share hospitals increased by $524,703.5. Although the increase after TennCare for DSHs is greater than that for non-DSHs, the graph on Figure 3 shows that there was an outlier in profit for DSHs in 1996. When this outlier is taken out then the median increase in profit after TennCare is not as great. The non-disproportionate share hospitals served as controls and they showed overall better financial performance after TennCare than the disproportionate-share hospitals. But the null hypothesis of same or decreased financial performance of disproportionate-share hospitals after TennCare implementation was accepted mainly due to the fact that the regression analysis showed that the hospitals had a positive B value prior to TennCare and a negative post-policy value afterwards.

When considering the financial performance of non-DSHs after TennCare implementation, it could be seen from table 5 that the hospitals had a net decrease of $4,942.51 per year. Although this represents a yearly loss in profit for non-DSHs, it is significantly better than the yearly loss of $45,319.4 sustained by the DSHs after TennCare implementation.

The second null hypothesis was that disproportionate-share hospitals will experience a decrease or no change in average daily census. Although the data analysis showed that median average daily census of DSHs decreased after TennCare implementation, the null hypothesis was not accepted. This is because regression analysis shows that the decrease in average median daily census prior to TennCare implementation was much greater than the decrease after TennCare. So after implementation of TennCare there was a decrease in linear downward trend. The regression analysis also showed that prior to TennCare, DSHs had a downward linear trend and were losing patients at an average of 3 patients per year. But after TennCare, average daily census was decreasing by only about 1 patient per year. That is an improvement over the trend that was occurring before TennCare implementation. When the graph of median average census was plotted against years for both DSHs and non-DSHs (figure 1), it could be observed that the downward trend of the graph decreased after TennCare implementation. Thus looking at the graph, there was a downward linear trend which if it had continued after TennCare implementation would have resulted in a significant decrease in median average daily census by 1998. But the downward trend as mentioned before decreased and this was especially noticeable after 1994. In other words, the rate of decrease in median average daily census was higher prior to TennCare implementation than after. It could thus be argued that without TennCare implementation there would have been a greater decrease in average daily census, but that the implementation of TennCare checked the decrease and then stabilized it. Thus the null hypothesis of same or decreased average census was rejected. On the other hand average daily census for non-DSHs was a net increase of .5 after TennCare implementation.

When comparing the median average daily census of DSHs and non-DSHs it could be observed that overall DSHs performed better under TennCare than non-DSHs. This is because prior to TennCare DSHs were losing more patients but after TennCare the rate of loss decreased significantly. Non-DSHs, on the other hand were losing just .5 patients per year and after TennCare there was a net increase of .5 patients per year.

The third null hypothesis stated that TennCare implementation would result in same or decreased hospital admissions (Discharges and Admissions). The null hypothesis was rejected. This is because regression analysis shows that the effect of TennCare implementation is a decrease of 5 patients per year. This is a definite improvement over the former decrease of 64.5 prior to TennCare implementation. Table 8 of discharges and admissions, also showed that average median discharges and admissions for DSHs increased by 111.5 after TennCare implementation. The graph of median discharges/admission plotted against years also indicate that while there were no statistically identifiable trends, median discharges and admissions were generally higher after TennCare implementation. Thus the null hypothesis of same or decreased hospital admissions after TennCare implementation was rejected.

When considering the regression analysis of non-DSHs it could be seen that the effect of TennCare on non-DSHs was a net increase of 45 per year. So overall discharges/admissions were better for non-DSHs than for DSHs after TennCare implementation. But both DSHs and non-DSHs saw improvements in their median discharges/admissions after TennCare implementation.

Generally disproportionate share hospitals did well under TennCare as far as average daily census and discharges/admissions were considered, and so did nondisproportionate share hospitals. But both groups of hospitals did not fare well when financial performance was considered after TennCare implementation.

The results of this study should be interesting both to health care policy makers and individuals interested in health care issues, as well as to students and practitioners of healthcare administration, public management and political science. It should also be interesting to different constituent groups that were opposed to TennCare's implementation. For instance, part of the argument of the Tennessee Hospital Association (THA) in its opposition to TennCare was based on the groups' apprehension that with unlimited enrollment to TennCare (as was previously planned), there would be a concurrent increase in cost shifting to other insurers as well as an increase in the amount or number of charity care provided.[238] The THA wanted the state to prove that the capitation rate for TennCare was going to be enough for the amount and variety of services to be provided.[239] The basis of this argument was that TennCare implementation would help bring about an increase in charity care and poorer financial performance of providers in general. But when the results of data analysis pertaining to financial performance of hospitals are considered it would appear that actually TennCare implementation was not as detrimental as feared, despite the fact that after TennCare there was an overall decrease in profit for disproportionate-share hospitals. This should be of interest especially since DSHs are most likely the hospitals which would treat a larger percentage of indigent or charity care patients. In other words DSHs are most likely to be considered safety net hospitals and one would expect higher loss in profit.

A growing number of Medicaid patients are now receiving their medical care within a managed care system.[240] Andrew Bindman et al, studied the effects on safety-net clinics of running Medicaid (Medi-Cal) as a managed care program in California. The basis of the study was whether or not safety net providers could maintain their share of Medicaid patients after implementation of mandatory Medi-Cal managed care in several of California's different counties.[241] Initially it appeared that the majority of California's safety net primary clinics had experienced a decline in the percentage of their patients insured by Medi-Cal. But after the overall decline in the number of Medi-Cal beneficiaries was controlled for, it became apparent that increased penetration of MediCal managed care in a particular county was not independently associated with a decline in the clinics' share of Medi-Cal patients.[242] This finding could be contrasted with the findings from this study on TennCare. The implementation of TennCare did not appear to actively decrease utilization and admission levels of DSHs. Despite the fact that the null hypothesis (which states that DSHs will experience same or decreased profit under TennCare) was accepted, the overall decrease in profit was not as big as was anticipated. In fact the profit of DSHs for some of the years after TennCare implementation appeared to have increased slightly.

It is also important to note that patient utilization (as measured by average daily census and discharges/admissions) improved after TennCare implementation, especially considering the fact that inpatient activity at community hospitals has fallen.[243] This is mostly because treatments and procedures that would have required inpatient stay a decade ago are now routinely delivered in outpatient settings, due to advancements in technology which allow for less invasive procedures that require less recuperation time. Increased availability of home health services and changes in reimbursement incentives have also contributed to declining hospital admissions. The decline in hospital admissions was most felt within rural hospitals. Admissions to urban hospitals were mostly flat from 1987 to 1993, while admissions to rural community hospitals continued to drop steadily.[244] From 1993 through 1997, USA hospital admissions increased very slightly (table 11).[245]

Table 11. Hospital Utilization and Revenue for the USA for Years 1993-1997

Years	1997	1998	1999	2000	2001
Admissions	31,047,930	30,652,820	30,577,564	30,403,766	30,475,563
Total Net Revenue (millions)	$322,460	$310,513	$298,520	$285,858	$274,526

This trend could also be contrasted with the rate of change of hospital admissions for Tennessee prior to and after implementation of TennCare. This comparison is done to determine if the changes noted for discharges/admissions for DSHs were mainly due to TennCare implementation instead of a reflection of what was going on at the national level. The graph for median discharges and admissions as mentioned before indicated that there was a downward trend, which then reversed and started increasing at about the time TennCare was implemented. Since this does not exactly mirror the trend that was going on at the national level, there is a greater degree of confidence in stating that the difference at the state level would largely be attributed to TennCare.

At the national level on the other hand, according to Hospital Statistics, there was an upward trend in outpatient visits as opposed to the downward trend in inpatient admissions. This was due mainly to both increased volume of surgical procedures being done on an outpatient basis and on substantial growth in number and variety of outpatient services provided by these hospitals.[246] When this national upward trend in outpatient visits was contrasted with data for Tennessee both before and after TennCare, it was clear that average daily census for hospitals in the state both before and after the reform program, did not follow the national trend. Rather than being on an upward trend, average daily census for the state showed a decline prior to TennCare but after the program, the downward trend appeared to have slightly leveled off.

Hospital financial trends have been affected by varying changes in hospital reimbursement policies, medical practice patterns, medical technology and social and market forces.[247] For the period spanning 1989 through 1992, yearly net revenue growth averaged about 11 percent, but 1993 growth was only about 6.7 percent. From 1993 through 1997, national hospital net revenue increased only slightly each respective year (table 11). The slowdown in revenue growth at the national level could be attributed to penetration of managed care networks, capitation and various other payment arrangements that fix in advance the amount of reimbursement a hospital will receive for a patient's care.[248] With less care being delivered on a fee for service basis, it was necessary for hospitals to try to ensure efficient delivery of services so as to better assure their solvency.

For the state of Tennessee, DSHs experienced moderate increases in profit while non-DSHs experienced marginal increases in profit during the period prior to TennCare implementation. After implementation of the reform program, for DSHs, there was a scattered trend in profit, with the overall effect of generating negative data analysis result for the post-TennCare variable. Median profit appeared to have increased for non-DSHs right after TennCare implementation after which there was a gradual decrease in profit.

Although the null hypothesis (which states that disproportionate-share hospitals will experience same or decreased profit after TennCare implementation) was accepted, further research is still needed to verify the long lasting effects of TennCare implementation on DSHs.

The results of this research are quite interesting considering that media portrayal of TennCare has been quite negative. The overwhelming negative portrayal of TennCare focused on the low reimbursement rates and on the possibility that these low rates would make it difficult for providers to break even. But this study's findings indicate that the negative portrayal should not be taken at face value, especially when considering the fact that TennCare provided insurance for individuals who otherwise would not have had insurance or who were uninsurable. The process of providing insurance for these individuals should at least lessen the burden of hospitals that would have had to provide charity care for these patients. The argument that TennCare has low reimbursement rates should be considered in conjunction with the fact that managed care systems basically have lower reimbursement rates for their providers, and TennCare is not an exception in that regard. Obviously parts of structural implementation of the program remain to be straightened out. The program has yet to be fine tuned so as to achieve the fullest possible benefits. Since the strategy for implementation was speedy in nature, there were problems working out the logistics of the program. It is not clear what if any effects this had on the data or results of the data analyses.

Limitations of the Study

These findings should be interpreted within possible limitations to the study. As mentioned, this study utilized the entire population of hospitals within the state of Tennessee, and as such the problems relating to its validity and confidence in its use are few but unique. The study results may have relevance for other states, although states differ in their administration and management of their Medicaid or managed care programs. The research is not really subject to validity issues since validity issues have to deal with measurement instruments and inferential statistics, but there could be possible questions of validity relating to the self reporting done by the hospitals or their administrators. There might have been some elements of misrepresentation in the self reporting by the administrators, though this is rather doubtful since they were providing this information for the state for record purposes. But it should also be borne in mind that a few of the hospitals did not follow the accounting principles enumerated by the state for the purposes of completing their financial information.

Another concern is the fact that some hospitals did not provide information on some of the variables on some years. But this should not be considered a major problem to confidence in the findings since the classified missing variables were very few in number.

It is also important to clarify that time series analysis usually incorporates a longer time span both before and after the independent variable interruption. That is, the years before and after the interruption are usually longer than 5 years so as to allow sufficient time to determine a consistent pattern or trend or to build a model for fluctuations. This is a possible limitation of the study. But overall, the study should be considered a valid analysis of the effects of TennCare reimbursement on disproportionate share hospitals, for the period spanning five years after the initial implementation of TennCare..

Implications for Public Policy

This study provides insight into the effects of managed care reimbursement on hospitals that serve a disproportionate number of indigent patients. Disproportionate share hospitals are part and parcel of the health care delivery system, but DSHs are unique in that they also act as safety net providers for uninsured patients who could not afford health care. As such they tend to provide care for a larger number of indigent patients than other hospitals. It is important then to determine if such hospitals can hold their own, especially when faced with the reality of managed care, particularly its conservative payment schema. The study was conducted to determine how a state mandated managed care schema affected utilization and financial well being of hospitals in general. As can be determined by the study, managed care implementation does not automatically mean decreased revenues nor decreased utilization of health care services. In fact, managed care organizations focus mainly on preventive services for their enrollees so that the enrollees would be healthier individuals. I the long run, this benefits the organizations since they do not have to cover expensive preventable diseases. Managed care enrollment could conceivably produce greater outpatient utilization but fewer inpatient stays. This could be one of the reasons for the slackening downward trend of average median daily census prior to TennCare implementation.

There has been an increase in managed care penetration throughout the United States. This increased penetration is driven by increasing health care costs and the quest to provide health insurance for a greater number of people. The majority of states are exploring new and inventive ways of cutting down on their health care costs while at the same time trying to provide coverage for an increasing number of individuals. Since "Creative Financing" techniques are no longer viable means of boosting state coffers and offsetting increased health care costs, different states are experimenting with different reform programs or moving towards enactment of reform programs. According to Bindman et al., most states as well as a substantial proportion of Medi-Cal (California Medicaid) beneficiaries have changed or are in the process of changing from a program of traditional fee-for-service (FFS) reimbursement to managed care plan enrollment.[249] The TennCare example should be thoroughly analyzed so that states on the brink of reform can learn from it and precisely determine the routes that their reform programs would take.

This study is important both to policy makers and public administration. Policy makers set the course for this reform program and policy makers as well as public administrators will help achieve change for other states that chose to reform the way that their state Medicaid programs are administered. The health care delivery system of any nation is of great importance to policy makers, and this is especially true in the United States, where health care issues drive policy. For example the push by breast cancer activists in United States of America, has led to greater amounts of money being allocated for funding in breast cancer research. The same is true for other diseases such as AIDS, multiple sclerosis etc. Since public administrators enforce or administer policy, research dealing with health care policy should be of importance to public administrators.

Implications for Future Research

This study is one of a number of empirical studies that deal with the effects of managed care program on providers, but it is the only one that has specifically dealt with determining the effects of TennCare on disproportionate share hospitals. The study by Bindman et al., can be considered one of a few studies that closely resemble this particular study. Bindman et al., tried to determine the effects of Medicaid managed care's impact on safety net clinics in California.[250] Safety net clinics can be considered similar to DSHs, because they cater to a larger percentage of indigent patients. The authors found that when the overall decline in the number of Medi-Cal beneficiaries was controlled for, the increased penetration of Medi-Cal managed care in a county was not correlated or associated with a decline in clinics' share of Med-Cal patients.[251]

The results from this study parallel the above in that most of the indicators show that as far as DSHs are concerned, managed care implementation might not be so detrimental to utilization and possibly financial performance. Table 5, which shows median profit for both DSHs and non-DSHs indicate that on the whole the profit of DSHs were higher after TennCare than previously. So TennCare implementation is possibly not as adverse to hospitals in Tennessee as media portrayals would indicate. Though the regression analysis does not support rejecting the null hypothesis, there is need for further research to explore if in the long run, TennCare implementation has an adverse effect on the profit of DSHs. Future studies could also look at profit as a percentage of revenue to see if the decrease in profit is due to decreased revenue or decreased efficiency on the whole. Further investigation can focus on the effects of specific or individual states' managed care programs on hospitals and especially disproportionate share hospitals. There is also room for replication of this study, especially in a few years to see if there are any lasting effects on DSHs. Future research efforts need to focus on possible ways of modifying the program's management to derive better benefits. This should be of importance especially since TennCare was implemented so hastily that there was really no time for ironing out the details of the reform plan, such as enrollment policies and provider selection. Other research areas could also focus on the quality of services delivered by TennCare.

Current State of TennCare, Future Implications and Conclusions

The state of Tennessee has seen two governors take office since TennCare was implemented. The state is currently under the governorship of Bredesen, who succeeded Governor Sundquist as the Governor of Tennessee. Both Governors cumulatively instituted many sweeping changes to TennCare program in an effort to cut the rising cost of the program. The majority of the changes started in 2000, when the program began to unravel. There were continuing problems with management of the program, high turnover of TennCare managerial positions as well as problems with Blue Cross of Tennessee. In addition providers became increasingly reluctant to accept new TennCare patients, especially since the payments for services rendered were not guaranteed. By the beginning of 2002, TennCare was consuming about 26% of the state's budget and the growing consensus was that the program should be scaled back. Then in 2002, when the Section 1115 waiver was renewed, the federal government backed out of contributing to the cost of expansion of coverage. As a result of the waiver, financial eligibility levels had been lowered for TennCare, resulting in thousands of premium paying people being dropped from the TennCare rolls, and there has been the implementation of a redetermination process that is user unfriendly resulting in the dis-enrollment of actually eligible people. The state has also instituted major reductions or elimination of coverage for citizens with chronic diseases.

Governor Bredesen announced on January, 2005, that part and parcel of his TennCare reform plan would result in the termination of coverage for adults on TennCare Standard[252] and TennCare Spend Down. By the first week of June, 2005, about 200, 000 adults that were on TennCare Standard had received letters notifying them that they were no longer eligible for TennCare standard but they should submit application for TennCare Medicaid. Termination letters for TennCare Spend down enrollees were slated to be sent out towards the later part of June 2005.[253]

Currently TennCare will no longer cover the following:

- Adults who were previously covered as uninsurable or medically eligible;
- Adults that have Medicare but do not receive Supplemental Security Income (SSI);
- Adults that were previously covered because they had catastrophic medical bills and thus were able to qualify for Medicaid Spend Down (Medicaid Spend Down or Medically Needy coverage allows people with catastrophically high medical bills get on TennCare. Prior to April, 29, 2005, people older than 65, the blind, the disabled and single parents were considered, but currently only children and pregnant women are considered).[254]

The following will still be eligible for TennCare Medicaid coverage:

- Children under 21;
- Pregnant women;
- Families that were on Families First[255]
- Individuals that receive SSI check
- Women currently on treatment for breast or cervical cancer
- Individuals that live in nursing homes with a monthly income that is below $1,373, or receives long-term care services that are paid for by TennCare;
- Individuals who stopped receiving SSI since November 13, 1987, while still living in Tennessee;
- Individuals who had previously received SSI and Social Security Check together at least once in the same month since April, 1977 and who still currently receive Social Security Check.[256]

The last chapter has not yet been written with regards to the bold and innovative TennCare program instituted by the State of Tennessee. There are still continuing changes to TennCare and only time will tell if the program will manage to survive or if it will be completely scraped and the State return to it Medicaid days. But one universal consensus is that in its hey days the program provided health insurance coverage to more people in Tennessee than were ever covered in recent decades by Medicaid, it did that while reigning in costs and expanding coverage and at the same time dealing with managerial issues pertaining to its implementation. .

The examination of effects of TennCare reimbursement on utilization and financial performance of disproportionate share hospitals is a central component of this book. The DSHs hospitals generally performed better than expected, especially considering the fact that media portrayal of TennCare had been so negative. DSHs managed to curb the downward trend in average median daily census after TennCare implementation. Median admissions and discharges actually went up generally after the reform program. The regression analysis on profit does not support rejecting the null hypothesis. Two of the null hypotheses[257] were rejected. The null hypothesis that states same or decreased profit for DSHs after TennCare implementation was accepted for this study. Further research and replication need to be carried out both for Tennessee as well as for other states with similar reform programs to determine if implementation of managed care and more comprehensive insurance coverage with better management could actually benefit DSHs and hospitals in general. This could help determine the focus of future health care policy in the United States. There is also the necessity for future research that focus on the managerial aspects of TennCare. Perhaps if the program had been better managed it could have been more successful and not be beset with so many problems. It might have even provided a workable blue print for the rest of the nation as far as universal provision of coverage is concerned.

Endnotes

Chapter 1

1 OECD stands for Organization for Economic Cooperation and Development.

2 OECD Health Data 1998, "A Comparative Analysis of 29 Countries,"(CD-ROM) (Paris: Organization for Economic Cooperation and Development, 1998).

3 Ibid

4 Sheila Smith, Mark Freeland, Stephen Heffler, David McKusick, Health Expenditures Projection Team, "The Next Ten Years of Health Spending: What Does the Future Hold?" Health Affairs (Millwood) 5, no. 17 (1998): 128-140.

5 R. Torrens, "Historical Evolution of Health Services in the United States," in Stephen J. Williams and Paul R. Torrens, ed., Introduction to Health Services, 4h Edition (New York: Delmar Publishers INC. 1993), 14-28.

6 Ibid

7 According to Paul Torrens, these Blue Cross and Blue shield plans were developed by hospital and physician associations, so as to spread health care costs more widely amongst the population.

8 Torrens, 14-28

9 Ibid

10 Thomas Bodenhimer and Kevin Grumbach, "The Reconfiguration of US Medicine" The Journal of The American Medical Association (JAMA) 274, no. 1 (July 5, 1995): 85-92.

11 Ibid

12 Ibid

13 Ibid

14 Ibid.

15 It is necessary to mention that individuals are ultimately the payers of all health care because individuals finance both government and businesses by paying taxes and purchasing the products of businesses.

16 Some insurers can also be considered as payers due to the fact that they can also pay for services while also being able to receive money from payers. The government can be viewed in this category when the Medicaid and Medicare programs are considered.

17 Bodenhimer and Grumbach

18 Thomas Kuhn, The Structure of Scientific Revolutions, 3rd ed. (The University of Chicago Press, 1970), 77-91

19 Kuhn, 84-85

20 This is a prospective reimbursement schema whereby health care providers are paid on a predetermined rate or a fixed dollar amount based on diagnosis of the condition being treated. As such diseases are classified into different categories with different payment levels for the different categories of diseases. If the diagnosis is for a cold for instance and the payment rate for that is say $50, then a provider could not be paid more than $50 regardless of cost of providing care to a particular patient that had the cold.

21 Torrens, 14-28.

22 Alma Koch, "Financing Health Services," in Stephen J. Williams and Paul R. Torrens, ed., Introduction to Health Services. 4th (New York: Delmar Publishers INC. 1993), 302.

23 Social Security Administration, "Social Security Programs in the United States," Social Security Bulletin 56, no. 4 (Washington, D.C.: U.S. Department of Health and Human Services, Winter 93).

24 Alma Koch, 311

25 Richard Rognehaugh, "The Managed Health Care Dictionary," 2nd ed. (Gaithersburg, Maryland: Aspen Publishers, Inc., 1998).

26 Alma Koch, 311-312.

27 Ibid

28 Ibid

29 Ibid

30 Social Security Administration, Social Security Bulletin. 1994 Supplement Statistics (Washington, D.C.: U.S. Department of Health and Human Services), 83.

31 This implies that medical services are provided as a welfare benefit instead of cash.

32 Alma Koch, 313.

33 Social Security Administration

34 Alma Koch, 309

35 Ibid; Milton I. Roemer, Social Medicine: The Advance of Organized Health Services in America (New York: Springer, 1978).

36 Drew Altman and Beatrice Dennis, "Perspectives on the Medicaid Program," Health Care Financing Review 12 (1990, Annual Supplement): 2-5.

37 HMOS utilize medical gatekeepers to ration the use of health care services. These gatekeepers are usually primary care physicians, and they have inbuilt incentives to ration medical care according to HMO's guidelines. This is depending on the particular HMO, the physicians' financial compensations are better when they keep within the HMO guidelines. The covered individual can switch HMOs if the guidelines are not acceptable, but the HMOs' guidelines are mostly determined by the premiums, i.e HMOs that have more costly premiums usually have more lax rationing rules. This idea is inherent in utilizing managed care for TennCare.

38 According to Health Care Financing Administration (HCFA), disproportionate share hospitals are described as those hospitals that serve a significantly disproportionate share of low income patients. In the 1999 issue of "Profiles of U.S. Hospitals," the measure that is used to determine the number of low income patients is the sum of two ratios: 1) Number of inpatient days that can be attributable to Medicare beneficiaries who also get federal supplementary security income (SSI) payments, as a proportion of total Medicare inpatient days, and 2) number of Medicaid inpatient days, considered as a proportion of total inpatient days. According to Association of American Medical Colleges, the DSH percentage varies with regards to size and geography of the hospital, for instance urban hospitals with more than 100 beds (which are usually the largest category of hospitals that receive disproportionate share payments) have a lower threshold of DSH percentage than rural area hospitals with less than 100 beds. Although varying formulae are used, it is important to note that once a specified DSH percentage threshold is attained, a more generous formula is then utilized, for calculating increased DSH payment adjustment.

39 Health Care Investment Analysts, Profiles of U.S Hospitals (Health Care Investment Analysts, Inc., Baltimore, Md., 1999). It is also important to note that according to the 1999 issue of "Profiles of U.S. hospitals," there are more than 1,700 disproportionate share hospitals in the United States.

40 John K. Inglehart, "Health Policy Report: Health Care Reform by the States," Journal of Medicine 330, no. 1(January 6 1994): 75-79.

41 Ibid; Wendy Mariner, "Problems with Employer-Provided Health Insurance: The Employee Retirement Income Security Act and Health Care Reform," New England Journal of Medicine 327 (1992): 1682-1685; State of Hawaii, "The Hawaii Prepaid Health Care Act" Hawaii Revised Statistical Section 393: 1-53

42 Ibid

43 Ned McWherter, "TennCare: A New Direction in Health Care" (Nashville: State of Tennessee Report), 1993.

44 Ibid

45 Gordon Bonneyman, "Status of TennCare" (Nashville, Tennessee: Center for Health Care Strategies, May, 1996).

46 General Accounting Office, "State and Local Finances: Some Jurisdictions Confronted by Short and Long Term Problems (Washington, D.C.: General Accounting Office, 1990 GAO/HRO-93-46).

47 McWherter

48 Jerry Cromwell, Killard W. Adamache, Carol Ammering, William J. Bartosch, Ann Boulis, "Equity of the Medicaid Program to the Poor Versus Taxpayers,' Health Care Financing Review 16 (1995): 75-104

49 According to Cromwell et al. in "Equity of the Medicaid Program to the Poor Versus Taxpayers." The standard for Tennessee Aid to Families with Dependent Children (AFDC) program is lower than that for 46 other states in the union.

50 General Accounting Office, "State and Local Finances: Some Jurisdictions Confronted by Short and Long Term Problems (Washington, D.C.: General Accounting Office, 1990 GAO/HRO-93-46)

51 McWherter

52 Ibid

53 Ibid

54 Bonneyman, in "Status of TennCare," indicated that the normal lack of medical care often culminated in increased emergency room visits for ailments that sometimes were not critical in nature.

55 Bonneyman

56 Chevy Chase, "Changing State and Federal Payment Policies for Medicaid Disproportionate-Share Hospitals," Health Affairs, May/June 1998.

57 Teresa Coughlin and David Liska, "The Medicaid Disproportionate Share Hospital Payment Program: Background and Issues," (Number A-14, in Series-New Federalism: Issues and Options for States), The Urban Institute 1999.

58 Ibid.

59 Chase

60 Ibid

61 Prior to enactment of the law, Tennessee as well as several other states in United States had managed to curb escalating health care costs by the use of "Creative Financing techniques, such as disproportionate-share hospital (DSH) payment subsidies as well as other enhanced provider payments.

62 The term "held harmless," as far as DSH payments are concerned, indicate that the providers that paid these taxes or that provided the donations were not going to be harmed financially." In other words they were at least going to get back the initial amount that they had donated or paid as taxes. But with this 1991 law, providers could no longer be guaranteed DSH payments that were at least equal to their taxes or donations. So taxes had to be "real assessments' and donations had to be "bonafide."

63 L. Ku and Teresa Coughlin, "Medicaid Disproportionate Share and Other Special Financing Programs," Health Care Financing Review 16, no.3 (1995): 1-54.

64 Terese Hudson, "States Scramble for Solutions Under New Medicaid Law," Hospitals 66, no. 11 (June, 1992): 52-55

65 Chase

66 Sidney D. Watson, "Medicaid Physician Participation: Patients, Poverty, and Physician Self Interest," American Journal of Law and Medicine no. 42 (1995): 142-151.

67 Coughlin and Liska.

68 Ibid

69 Ibid

70 Chase

71 In William Cleverly, Essentials of Health Care Finance (Rockville, MD. Aspen Systems Corporation, 1978), 134-158. This can refer to indirect medical education adjustment or allowance that is given to a teaching hospital. This allowance is related to the hospital bed size as well as the number of interns and residents at the hospital. The allowance is usually over and above salaries paid to interns and residents. The adjustment is meant to cover the additional costs incurred by the teaching hospital in the treatment of patients. Hospitals that treat a large percentage of Medicare and Medicaid patients also get a separate payment. This payment is referred to as the disproportionate payment.

72 Hudson

73 Inter-government transfers are fund exchanges between or among different levels of government, such as state or county governments.

74 Chase

75 Ibid

76 Coughlin and Liska.

77 Ibid

78 Chase

79 Ibid

80 Ku and Coughlin, 1-54.

81 Coughlin and Liska.

82 Before any state can reform the way it's Medicaid program is administered, it has to obtain a research and demonstration waiver from HCFA. HCFA is the federal agency that is in charge of administering Medicare and overseeing states' administration of Medicaid. The organization is also responsible for publishing reports on plan performance and reviewing Medicare HMO applications. (Richard Rognnehaugh, "The Managed Health Care Dictionary," Gaithersburg, Maryland: Aspen Publishers, Inc., 1998, 2rid ed.).

83 Sandy Lutz, "For Real Reform, Watch The States," Modern Healthcare 25, no.4 (1995): 30-33

84 Ibid

85 Ibid

86 Bonneyman

Endnotes 79

87 David M. Mirivis, Cyril F. Chang, Christopher J. Hall, Gregory T. Zaar, William B. Applegate, "TennCare: Health System Reform for Tennessee," Journal of the American Medical Association. 274, no.15 (October 18, 1995): 1235.

88 McWherter.

89 Ibid

90 Ibid

91 Elizabethann O'Sullivan and Gary Rassell, Research Methods for Public Administrators, 2nd ed. (White Plains, New York: Longman Publishers, 1995), 69.

92 Office of Health Statistics, (Joint Annual Hospital Reports), Tennessee Department of Health (1989-1998). The data collected by TDH includes amongst others, information pertaining to average daily census, indigent charges adjustment, Medicaid, Medicare and TennCare profit, admissions/discharges, operating and non-operating revenue sources and patient origin.

93 William Cleverly, 134-158.

94 Aaron Katz and Jack Thompson, 'The Role of Public Policy in Health Care Market Change," Health Affairs 15, no. 2 (Summer, 1996): 77-79.

95 Ibid

96 Scott MacStravic, "Market Memo: Managing Utilization:The Old Way and The New Way," Health Care Strategic Management, (October, 1996).

97 Katz and Thompson, 77-79.

98 Guy B. Peters, American Public Policy: Promise and Performance 3rd ed., (Chatham. N.J.: Chatham House, 1993).

99 Randall Ripley and Grace Franklin, Congress. the Bureaucracy. and Public P Policy Revised ed., (Homewood, Ill: Dorsey Press. 1987).

100 Thomas R. Dye. Understanding Public Policy 5th ed. (Englewood Cliffs, New Jersey: Prentice-Hall, 1984).

101 Gregg S. Meyer and David Blumenthal, "TennCare and Academic Medical Centers: The Lessons from Tennessee," Journal of the American Medical Association 276, no. 9 September 1994): 672-677

102 Charles R. Fisher, "Trends in Total Hospital Financial Performance Under the Prospective Payment System," Health Care Financing Review 13, no. 3 (Spring 1992).

103 Denise M. McCollum, "The Structural Response and Performance of General Hospitals in a Managed Care Environment," (Ph.D. Dissertation, Virginia Commonwealth University) Feb 1999.

104 Cynthia A. Hatton, "Effects of Medicare Reimbursement on Home Health Care. (Master of Science Dissertation, San Jose State University) Fall 1990.

105 John J. Harrington, "Medicaid and Managed Care: An Implementation Study of the Tennessee Primary Care Network," (Ph.D. Dissertation, Brandeis U., The F. Heller Graduate School For Advanced Studies in Social Welfare) Nov 1996.

106 Darrell J. Gaskin, "The Impact of Health Maintenance Organization Penetration on the use of Hospitals that Serve Minority Communities," Medical Care 35 no. 12 (1997): 1190-1203.

107 MacStravic

Chapter 2

108 Ibid

109 Tennessee Public Acts of 1993.

110 Gordon Bonneyman, "Status of TennCare" (Nashville, Tennessee: Center for Health Care Strategies, May, 1996).

111 McWherter, "TennCare: A New Direction in Health Care," Nashville State of Tennessee Report 1993

112 Allen Dobson, Donald Moran, Gary J. Young, "The Role of Federal Waivers in the Health Policy Process," Health Affairs 11, no. 4 (1993): 72-94; Jerry Cromwell, Killard W. Adamache, Carol Ammering, William J. Bartosch, Ann Boulis, "Equity of the Medicaid Program to the Poor Versus Taxpayers," Health Care Finance Review 16, (1995): 75-104.

113 United States Bureau of the Census, Statistical Abstract of the United States. (Washington, D.C.: U.S. Government Printing Office, 1999).

114 Ibid

115 Ibid

116 Ibid

117 These cost containment measures parallel the measures found in President Clinton's health plan.

118 McWherter

119 National Association of Public Hospitals, "Assessing the Design and Implementation of TennCare." (Washington, D.C.: U.S. Government Printing Office, 1994).

120 Ibid

121 A Managed Care Organization (MCG), is a type of managed care plan similar to a Health Maintenance Organization

122 National Association of Pubic Hospitals.

123 Lauren Walker, "How not to Launch Health Reform," Medical Economics 72, no. 12 (June 26, 1995): 88-90.

124 Ibid

125 David M. Mirvis, Cyril F. Chang, Christopher J. Hall, Gregory T. Zaar, William B. Applegate, "TennCare: Health System Reform for Tennessee." Journal of American Medical Association 274, no.15 (October 18, 1995): 1235-1241.

126 These Managed Care Organizations (MCOs) are private, nonprofit health plans that are licensed by the state.

127 Walker

128 Mirvis et al., 1235-1241.

129 Ibid

130 HMO is described as a line of business that is focused on managing populations of patients through a prepaid premium, and selling this licensed product directly to the employer or purchaser. Under the federal HMO act, the organization must have three characteristics: an organized system for the provision of care or otherwise ensuring health care delivery in a geographic area, an agreed-on set of basic and supplemental health maintenance and treatment services and a voluntary enrolled group of patients. Richard Rognehaugh, "The Managed Health Care Dictionary," 2nd ed. (Gaithersburg, Maryland: Aspen Publishers Inc., 1998).

131 PPO is the term used to describe a plan or an affiliation of providers seeking contracts with a plan on the basis of their ability to cover a broad geographical area or

provide multi specialty skills. Richard Rognehaugh, "The Managed Health Care Dictionary," 2nd ed. (Gaithersburg, Maryland: Aspen Publishers Inc., 1998).

132 The Tennessee Primary Care Network was the only HMO serving Medicaid recipients before the implementation of TennCare.

133 PPOs usually pass the risk to their provider net works, and they might adjust
rates paid to providers if their payments are higher than the capitation payment they receive from the state. On the other hand, HMOs assume the financial risks for their
patients by guaranteeing rates to providers.

134 Mirvis et al., 1235-1241.

135 Ibid

136 McWherter.

137 Ibid

138 Ibid

139 See for example: Lauren Walker, "How not to Launch Health Reform." *Medical
Economics* 72, no.12 (June 26, 1995): 88; Cyril F. Chang, Laurel J. Kiser, James B. Bai-
ley, Manny Martins, William C. Gibson, Kari A. Schaberg, David M. Mirvis, William B.
Applegate, "Tennessee's Failed Managed Care Program for Mental Health and Substance
Abuse Services," JAMA, *Journal of the American Medical Association* 279, no.11
(March 18, 1998): 864-869.

140 National Association of Public Hospitals

141 Ibid

142 Ibid

143 National Association of Public Hospitals; Robert E. Hurley, Deborah A. Freund,
J. E. Paul, Managed Care in Medicaid: Lessons for Policy and Program Design (Ann
Arbor, Michigan: Health Administration Press, 1993)

144 Robert J. Blendon, Karen Donelan, Craig Hill, "Medicaid Beneficiaries and
Health Reform." *Health Affairs* (Millwood) no.12 (1993):132-143.

145 Guy B. Peters, *American Public Policy: Promise and Performance*, 3rd edition,
(Chatham, New Jersey: Chatham House, 1993).

146 Randall Ripley and Grace Franklin, *Congress, The Bureaucracy, and Public
Policy*, Revised ed. (Homewood, Ill: Dorsey Press, 1980).

147 Matthew Cahn, "The Players: Institutional and Noninstitutional Actors in the
Policy Process," in *Public Policy: The Essential Readings*, ed. Stella Theodoulou and
Matthew Calm (Englewood Cliffs, NJ: Prentice Hall, 1995), 201-211.

148 Ibid.

149 Stella Theodoulou. "The Nature of Public Policy" In *Public Policy: The Essential Readings*, ed. Stella Theodoulou and Matthew Calm (Englewood Cliffs, NJ: Prentice
Hall. 1995), 5.

150 Stella Theodoulou, "Making Public Policy," In *Public Policy: The Essential
Readings*, ed. Stella Theodoulou and Michael Calm (Englewood Cliffs, NJ: Prentice Hall,
1995), 86-87.

151 George C. Edwards III, *Implementing Public Policy* (Washington D.C.: Congressional Quarterly Press, 1980).

152 Stella Theodoulou, "Making Public Policy."

153 Ibid

154 Eugene Bardach, "The Implementation Gamer," in Public Policy: The Essential
Readings, ed. Stella Theodoulou and Michael Cahn (Englewood Cliffs, NJ: Prentice Hall,
1995), 137-139.

155 Paul Sabatier, Daniel Mazmanian, "A Conceptual Framework of the Implementation Process," in *Public Policy: The Essential Readings*, ed. Stella Theodoulou and Michael Cahn (Englewood Cliffs, NJ: Prentice Hall, 1995), 153-154.

156 Bonneyman

157 National Association of Public Hospitals.

158 Terese Hudson, "Vision of the Future: Tennessee Hospitals, Physicians Worry Over TennCare," *Hospitals and Health Networks* 68, no.7 (April 5, 1994): 44-47; Mirvis et al.

159 Mirvis et al.

160 Ibid

161 Ibid

162 Ibid

163 National Association of Public Hospitals.

164 It is important to note this point. The association probably had a valid case in point because the state of Tennessee announced its intent to drop 91,000 recipients who failed to pay premiums. The majority of these recipients did not receive their payment booklets from the state, and this was probably why they could not send in their premiums. The mistake could be attributed to inadequate accounting and data management systems. This scenario provides an example of the mismanagement and confusion that resulted due to fast implementation of the program.

165 TPN is a managed care program that is run by Blue Cross /Blue Shield of Tennessee.

166 Andrew Jackson Institute, "Effects of Formulary Restrictions on Patient Treatment: A Survey Among Physicians Enrolled in TennCare," (Nashville, Tennessee: Andrew Jackson Institute) 1994.

167 For instance, the consumer survey that was supposed to be conducted 6 months after the implementation of TennCare had not been reported and there were no well developed comprehensive management information systems.

168 McWherter

169 Paul Schulman, "Non-incremental Policy Making," In *Public Policy: The Essential Readings*, ed. Stella Theodoulou and Michael Cahn (Englewood Cliffs, NJ: Prentice Hall, 1995) 128.

170 National Association of Public Hospitals.

171 Mirvis et al.

172 National Association of Public Hospitals

173 These patients have diseases that are very expensive to treat or manage. Such diseases would include AIDS, hemophilia etc.

174 Mirvis et al.

175 National Association of Public Hospitals.

176 Mirvis et al.

177 Ibid

178 National Association of Public Hospitals.

179 Ibid

180 It is necessary to note that these were questionnaires that dealt with patients' perceptions of quality of service, and thus could not really serve as a true indicator of the

level or standard of medical care received by these patients. Generally only a doctor is fully qualified to make such a determination based on patient history and treatment.

181 Despite all these complaints there is no study yet that has conclusively shown that TennCare implementation (for the period spanning 1994 through 1998) has hampered the quality of care received by the majority of enrollees.

182 National Association of Public Hospitals.

183 Bonneyman

184 Ibid

185 National Association of Public Hospitals

186 Ibid

187 Ibid

188 Joseph Anthos, "Waivers, Research and Health System Reform," *Health Affairs* (Millwood) 12, no.1 (1993): 178-183.

189 The categorization for 100% poverty level determines that to be characterized as being on 100% poverty level the income should be $581 per month for a single individual or $1,196 for a family of 4.

190 McWherter

191 General Accounting Office, "Medicaid: States Turn to Managed Care to Improve Access and Control Costs." (Washington, D.C.: General Accounting Office, 1993 GAO/HRO-93-46).

192 Robert E. Hurley, Deborah Freund, J. E. Paul, "Managed Care in Medicaid." (AnnArbor, Michigan: Health Administration Press, 1993).

193 Jack Zwanziger, and Rebecca Averbach, "Evaluating PPO Performance Using Prior Expenditure Data." *Medical Care* 29 (1991): 142-151.

194 Bonneyman

195 Ibid

Chapter 3

196 Thomas Cook and Donald Campbell, *Ouasi-Experimentation: Design and Analysis Issues for Field Settings.* (Boston: Houghton Mifflin Company, 1979), 207.

197 Ibid

198 Ibid

199 Elizabeth O'Sullivan and Gary Rassell, *Research Methods for Public Administrators,* 2nd ed. (White Plains, New York: Longman Publishers, 1995), 69.

200 Cook and Campbell

201 Susan Welch and John Comer, *Quantitative Analysis in Public Administration: Techniques and Applications.* 2nd ed. (Pacific Grove, California, Brooks/Cole Publishing Company, 1988), 288-296.

202 *SPSS,* INC. *SPSS Base Application Guide.* Chicago: SPSS, Inc., 1998.

203 O'Sullivan and Rassell, 242.

204 Ibid

205 Tennessee Department of Health, *Joint Annual Report of Hospitals,* (Nashville, Tennessee: Office of Health Statistics, 1998).

206 The data on profit was adjusted to reflect the fact that a dollar in 1989 is not worth the same as a dollar in 1998. Inflation through the years would have eroded some of the value of the dollar. So all the dollar values for profit were transformed into standard dollar. This was achieved using the consumer prize index measure, which is found in yearly Statistical Abstract of the United States.

207 Association of American Medical Colleges. *Medicare Disproportionate Share* (DSH) *Payments* .http://www.aamc.org/advocacy/library/teachhosp/hosp0003.htm assessed, August 10 2006.

208 Ibid.

209 Provisions were made by Congress in OBRA 1993, so as to make it difficult for states to retain their disproportionate share payments instead of using the funds to make payments to DSH.

210 O'Sullivan and Rassell, 48-50.

211 Ibid

212 Welch and Coiner, 288.

213 Ibid

214 Ibid

215 Cook and Campbell, 211.

216 David Morgan and Kenneth Kickham, "Changing the Form of County Government: Effects on Revenue and Expenditure Policy," *Public Administration Review 59*, no. 4 (July/August 1999): 318.

217 Ibid

218 Ibid

219 Ibid

220 Ibid

221 Cook and Campbell, 213-214

222 Welch and Coiner, 288.

223 Ibid

224 Ibid

225 Ibid

226 Ibid

227 Ibid

228 Ibid

Chapter 4

229 Elizabeth O'Sullivan and Gary R Rassell, *Research Methods for Public Administrators*, 2nd ed. (White Plains, New York: Longman Publishers, 1995), 351-369.

230 Ibid

231 O'Sullivan and Rassell, 313-350.

232 Ibid

233 1t should be noted that interpreting the R square value is very complicated. A good rule of thumb in interpreting the values is that the closer to 1 the value is, the higher the confidence when interpreting the coefficients. For example an R square of .98 for average median daily census, indicates that 98% of the variation in the average median daily census can be "explained" using the linear regression model (which includes three variables). This simply means that this model should do a good job of predicting the observed medians. This high R square really measures how well separate lines for before and after TennCare fit the data. So it is more of a measure of the strength of linear trend over time than a measure of the effect of TennCare. So the high R square value will be utilized to argue that a good model is obtained, and thus the interpretations based on the regression coefficients carry more weight.

234 O'Sullivan and Rassell, 3 13-350

235 Ibid

236 The unstandardized coefficients are utilized statistically in quantifying the trend. Thus at zero B value, there is no trend and the farther away from zero the value, the steeper the trend.

237 The R square value for profit is not very close to one, thus the regression model does not fit that well. So interpretations of the coefficients should be made with more caution.

Chapter 5

238 Mirvis et al. "TennCare: Health System Reform for Tennessee," *Journal of the American Medical Association* 274, no.15 (October 18, 1995): 1235-1242.

239 Ibid

240 Andrew B. Bindman, Kevin Grumbach, Susannah Bernheim, Karen Vranizan, and Michael Cousineau, "Medicaid Managed Care's Impact on Safety-Net Clinics in California," *Health Affairs* 19 no.1 (Jan/Feb 2000).

241 Ibid

242 Ibid

243 Health Forum for American Hospital Association Company, *Hospital Statistics*, (One North Franklin Chicago: Illinois 60606-342, 1999 Edition).

244 Ibid

245 Ibid

246 Ibid

247 Ibid

248 Ibid

249 Bindman et al.

250 Ibid

251 Ibid

252 TennCare Standard is usually for individuals who could pay a monthly premium but were not eligible for TennCare Medicaid, though not everyone on TennCare standard could afford to pay a premium. These individuals are usually uninsured, uninsurable or medically ineligible, but effective April 29, 2005, adults over 19 are no longer eligible for TennCare Standard.

253 TennCare Information: Tennessee Alliance for Legal Services http://www.tals.org/publicweb/TennCare assessed August 6, 2006.

254 Ibid.

255 Families First is Tennessee's welfare reform plan that replaced the Aid to Families with Dependant Children (AFDC). The program offers temporary cash assistance but at the same time emphasizes work, training and personal responsibility. Thus participants are expected to wean (there are specific exceptions and exemptions) themselves off the program over a period spanning 18 months up to a maximum of lifetime assistance of 60 months.

256 TennCare Information, http://www.tals.org/publicweb/TennCare assessed August 6, 2006.

257 The two null hypotheses that were rejected are: 1) Hospitals that serve disproportionate number of low income people will experience negative or no improvement in financial performance under TennCare. 2) Disproportionate-share hospitals will experience a decrease or no change in average daily census.

Bibliography

Association of American Medical Colleges. *Medicare Disproportionate Share* (DSH) Payments.http://www.aamc.org/advocacy/library/teachhosp/hosp0003.htm assessed, August 10 2006.

American Hospital Association Company. *Hospital Statistics.* One North Franklin Chicago: Illinois 60606-342, 1999.

Andrew Jackson Institute. "Effects of Formulary Restrictions on Patient Treatment: A Survey Among Physicians Enrolled in TennCare." Nashville, Tennessee: Andrew Jackson Institute, 1994.

Altman, Drew and Beatrice Dennis. "Perspectives on the Medicaid Program." *Health Care Financing Review* 12 (1990, Annual Supplement): 2-5.

Antos, Joseph. "Waivers, Research and Health System Reform." *Health Affairs* (Millwood). 12, no.1 (1993): 178-183.

Bardach, Eugene. "The Implementation Game." In *Public Policy: The Essential Readings*, ed. Stella Theodoulou and Michael Cahn. Englewood Cliffs, New Jersey: Prentice Hall, 1995.

Bindman B. Andrew, Kevin Grumbach, Susannah Bernheim, Karen Vranizan, and Michael Cousineau. "Medicaid Managed Care's Impact on Safety-Net Clinics in California." *Health Affairs* 19, no.1 (January/February 2000).

Blendon, Robert, Karen Donelan, Craig Hill. "Medicaid Beneficiaries and Health Reform." *Health Affairs* (Millwood). 12 (1993): 132-143.

Bodenhimer, Thomas and Kevin Grumbach. "The Reconfiguration of United States Medicine." *Journal of The American Medical Association* 274, no.1 (July 5, 1995): 85-92.

Bonneyman, Gordon. "Status of TennCare." Nashville, Tennessee: Center for Health Care Strategies, (May 1996).

Cahn, Matthew. "The Players: Institutional and Non-institutional Actors in the Policy Process." In *Public Policy: The Essential Readings*, ed. Stella Theodoulou and Matthew Cahn. Englewood Cliffs, New Jersey: Prentice Hall, 1995.

Chang, F. Cyril, Laurel J. Kiser, James E. Bailey, Manny Martins, William Gibson. Kari A. Schaberg, David M. Mirvis, William B. Applegate. "Tennessee's Failed Managed Care Program for Mental Health and Substance Abuse Services. *Journal of the American Medical Association* 279, no.11 (March 18, 1998): 864-869

Chase, Chevy. "Changing State and Federal Payment Policies For Medicaid Disproportionate-Share Hospitals." *Health Affairs*, (May/June 1998).

Cleverly, William. *Essentials of Health Care Finance.* Rockville, MD: Aspen Systems Corporation, 1978.

Cook, Thomas and Donald Campbell. "Quasi-Experimentation: Design and Analysis Issues for Field Settings." Boston: Houghton Mifflin Company, 1979.

Coughlin, Teresa and David Liska. "The Medicaid Disproportionate-Share Hospital Payment Program: Background And Issues." Number A-14, in Series -New Federalism: Issues and Options For States. Washington D.C.: The Urban Institute, 1999.

Cromwell, Jerry, Killard Adamache, Carol Ammering, William Bartosch J. and Ann

A. "Equity of The Medicaid Program to The Poor Versus Taxpayers." *Health Care Financing Review* 16 (1995): 75-104.

Dobson Allen, Donald Moran and Gary Young. "The Role of Federal Waivers in the Health Policy Process." *Health Affairs* 11, no.4 (1993):72-94.

Dye, Thomas. *Understanding Public Policy.* Englewood Cliffs, New Jersey: Prentice Hall, 1984.

Edwards III, George. *Implementing Public Policy.* Washington D.C.: Congress Quarterly Press, 1980.

Fisher, R. Charles. "Trends in Total Hospital Financial Performance Under the Prospective Payment System." *Health Care Financing Review* 13, no. 3 (Spring 1992).

Gaskin, J. Darrell. "The Impact of Health Maintenance Organization Penetration on the Use of Hospitals that Serve Minority Communities." *Medical Care* 35, no. 12 (1997): 1190-1203.

General Accounting Office. "Medicaid: States Turn to Managed Care to Improve Access and Control Costs." Washington, D.C., 1993 (GAO/HRO-93-46).

General Accounting Office. State and Local Finance: Some Jurisdictions Confronted by Short and Long Term Problems." Washington, D.C., 1990 (GAO/HRO-93-46.

Harrington, J. John. "Medicaid and Managed Care: An Implementation Study of the Tennessee Primary Care Network." Ph.D. Dissertation, Brandeis U., The F, Heller Graduate School For Advanced Studies in Social Welfare, November, 1996.

Hatton A. Cynthia. "Effects of Medicare Reimbursement on Home Health Care." Master of Science Dissertation, San Jose State University, Fall, 1990.

Hawaii. "The Hawaii Prepaid Health Care Act. *Hawaii Revised Statistical Section.* 393.

Health Care Investment Analysts. *Profiles of U.S. Hospitals.* Baltimore, M.D.: Health Care Investment Analysts Inc., 1999.

Health Forum for American Hospital Association Company, *Hospital Statistics,* (One North Franklin Chicago: Illinois 60606-342, 1999 Edition).

Hudson, Terese. "States Scramble For Solutions Under New Medicaid Law." *Hospitals* 66, no.11 (June, 1992):52-55.

Hudson, Terese. "Vision of the Future: Tennessee Hospitals, Physicians Worry Over TennCare," *Hospitals and Health Networks* 68, no.7 (April 5, 1994): 44-47.

Hurley, Robert, Deborah Freund and J. E. Paul. *Managed Care in Medicaid: Lessons for Policy and Program Design.* Ann Arbor, Michigan: Health Administration Press, 1993.

Inglehart, John K. "Health Policy Report: Health Care Reform by The States." *Journal of Medicine* 330, no.1(January 6, 199): *75-79.*

Katz, Aaron and Jack Thompson. "The Role of Public Policy in Health Care Market Change." *Health Affairs* 15, no.2 (Summer, 1996): 77-79.

Koch, Alma. "Financing Health Services." In *Introduction to Health Services,* ed. Stephen J. Williams and Paul Torrens, New York: Delmar Publishers Inc., 1993, 4th ed.

Ku, L. and Teresa Coughuin. "Medicaid Disproportionate-Share And Other Special Financing Programs." *Health Care Financing Review* 16. no.3 (1995): 1-54.

Kuhn, Thomas. *The Structure of Scientific Revolutions.* 3rd ed. Chicago: University of Chicago Press, 1970.

Lutz, Sandy. "For Real Reform, Watch The States." *Modem Health Care 25,* no. 4 (1995): 30-33.

MacStravic, Scott. "Market Memo: Managing Utilization-The Old Way and The New Way." *Health Care Strategic Management.* (October, 1996).

Mariner, Wendy K. "Problems with Employee Retirement Income Security Act and Health Care *Reform.*" *New England Journal of Medicine* 327 (1992): 1682-1685

McCollum, M. Denise. "The Structural Response and Performance of General Hospitals in a Managed Care Environment." Ph.D. Dissertation, Virginia Commonwealth University, February, 1999.

McWherter, Ned. "TennCare: A New Direction in Health Care." *Nashville: State of Tennessee Report.* Nashville, TN (1993).

Meyer S. Gregg and David Blumenthal. "TennCare and Academic Medical Centers: The Lessons from Tennessee." *Journal of the American Medical Association* 276, no. 9 (September, 1994): 672-677.

Mirvis, M. David, Cyril F. Chang, Christopher J. Hall, Gregory T. Zaar, and William B Applegate. "TennCare: Health System Reform for Tennessee." *Journal of The American Medical Association* 274, no.15 (October 18, 1995): 1235-1242.

Morgan, David and Kenneth Kickham. "Changing the Form of County Government Effects on Revenue and Expenditure Policy." *Public Administration Review* 59, no. 4 (July/August 1999): 318.

National Association of Public Hospitals. "Assessing the Design and Implementation of TennCare." Washington, D.C.: National Association of Public Hospitals. 1994

OECD Health Data 1998, "A Comparative Analysis of 29 Countries," (Paris: Organization for Economic Cooperation and Development, 1998) CD-ROM

O'Sullivan, Elizabethann and Gary R. Rassell. *Research Methods for Public Administrators.* White Plains, New York: Longman Publishers USA. 1995

Peters, B. Guy. *American Public Policy: Promise and Performance*, 3rd ed.,Chatham.. New Jersey: Chatham House, 1993.

Richard, Rognehaugh, *"The Managed Health Care Dictionary,"* 2nd ed. (Gaithersburg, Maryland: Aspen Publishers Inc., 1998).

Ripley, Randall and Grace Franklin. *Congress. The Bureaucracy and Public Policy.* Revised edition, Homewood, Ill: Dorsey Press, 1980.

Roemer, Milton I. Social Medicine: *The Advance of Organized Health Services in America*, New York: Springer, 1978.

Sabatier, Paul and Daniel Mazmanian. "A Conceptual Framework of the Implementation Process." In *Public Policy: The Essential Readings*, ed. Stella Theodoulou and Michael Calm. Englewood Cliffs, New Jersey: Prentice Hall, 1995.

Schulman, Paul. "Non-incremental Policy Making.' In *Public Policy: The Essential Readings*, ed. Stella Theodoulou and Michael Cahn. Englewood Cliffs. New Jersey: Prentice Hall, 1995.

Smith, Sheila, Mark Freeland, Stephen Heffler and David McKusick of Health Expenditures Projection Team. "The Next Ten Years of Health Spending: What does The Future Hold?" *Health Affairs* (Millwood) 17, no.5 (1998): 128-140.

Social Security Administration. *Social Security Bulletin*, 1994 Supplement Statistics. Washington, D.C.: United States Department of Health and Human Services.

Social Security Administration. "Social Security Programs in The United States," *Social Security Bulletin* 56 no.4. Washington, D.C.: United States Department of Health and Human Services, 1993.

SPSS, Inc. *SPSS Base 8.0 Application Guide*. Chicago: SPSS, Inc., 1998.

Stella Theodoulou. "The Nature of Public Policy" In *Public Policy: The Essential Readings*, ed. Stella Theodoulou and Matthew Calm (Englewood Cliffs, NJ: Prentice Hall. 1995), 5.

Stella Theodoulou, "Making Public Policy," In *Public Policy: The Essential Readings*, ed. Stella Theodoulou and Michael Calm (Englewood Cliffs, NJ: Prentice Hall, 1995), 86-87.

Tennessee Department of Health. *Joint Annual Report of Hospitals*, Nashville TN: Office of Health Statistics, 1998.

Tennessee Public Acts of 1993.

Torrens, Paul R. "Historical Evolution of Health Services in the United States In *Introduction to Health Services* ed. Stephen J. Williams and Paul Torrens. New York: Delmar Publishers Inc., 1993.

United States Bureau of the Census, *Statistical Abstract of the United States*: Washington, DC: 1994.

United States Bureau of the Census, *Statistical Abstract of the United States*: Washington, DC: 1999.

Walker, Lauren. "How not to Launch Health Reform." *Medical Economics* 72. no 12 (June 26, 1995): 88-90.

Watson, Sidney D. "Medicaid Physician Participation: Patients, Poverty, And Physician Self Interest." *American Journal of Law And Medicine*, 42(1995): 142-151

Welch, Susan and John Comer. *Quantitative Analysis in Public Administration: Techniques and Applications*. 2nd ed. Pacific Grove, California: Brooks/Cole Publishing Company, 1988.

Zwanziger, Jack. and Averbach, R. "Evaluating PPO Performance Using Prior Expenditure Data.' *Medical Care*. 29 (1991): 142-151.

Index

About the Author

Chinyere Chigozie Ogbonna was born in Okwe, Nigeria. She completed her elementary education at Ekulu Primary School, Enugu in 1980. She graduated from Federal Government College, Enugu in 1985. She earned a Bachelor of Science Degree (Honors) in Parasitology and Entomology from Anambara State University, Enugu, Nigeria in 1990 and a Master of Science Degree in Health Care Administration from Western Kentucky University in 1996. Her Doctorate in Public Administration was earned at Tennessee State University in August 2000.

Dr Ogbonna has held various positions in both private and public health care industries, including research positions at Vanderbilt and Vectors /Arbovirus Research division under the auspices of World Health Organization and in 2001 she served as Bioterrorism Epidemiologist for Tennessee Department of Health.

Dr Ogbonna is currently employed as an Assistant Professor of Public Management at Austin Peay State University.

www.ingramcontent.com/pod-product-compliance
Lightning Source LLC
Chambersburg PA
CBHW021822270326
41932CB00007B/299